Joint and Soft Tissue Injection

injecting with confidence

Fifth Edition

Trevor Silver

MBBS (DUNELM), DA (RCS ENG), FRCGP

Contributing authors

David Silver

BSC, MBBS, FRCP (UK), FRCR

Consultant Radiologist

Royal Devon and Exeter Hospital

David MacLellan

Grad Dip Physio, Dip RG, RT, MCSP, HPC

Physiotherapist and Sports Medicine Specialist

Ocean Physiotherapy, Exeter

Radcliffe Publishing

London • New York

Radcliffe Publishing Ltd
33–41 Dallington Street
London
EC1V 0BB
United Kingdom

www.radcliffepublishing.com
Electronic catalogue and worldwide online ordering facility.

First edition 1996
Second edition 1999
Third edition 2002
Fourth edition 2007

British Library Cataloguing in Publication Data

A catalogue record for this book is available from the British Library.

ISBN-13: 978 1 84619 500 6

The paper used for the text pages of this book is FSC® certified. FSC (The Forest Stewardship Council®) is an international network to promote responsible management of the world's forests.

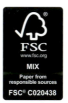

Typeset by Phoenix Photosetting, Chatham, Kent
Printed and bound by Hobbs the Printers Ltd, Totton, Hampshire

CONTENTS

PREFACE

In this book the author has provided a concise desk-top guide that will provide the practitioner with a comprehensive description and illustration for treatment of most common joint and soft tissue disorders that can be treated effectively in general practice. Medical education workshops organised by tutors are a good introduction to the subject, and realistic models (simulators) may be used as teaching aids to allow repeated practice of all the techniques a practitioner could wish to learn, thus avoiding the necessity of learning and practising on live patients. Models of the shoulder, wrist and hand, knee joint and elbow joint are available. These are marketed by Limbs and Things Ltd of Bristol and I acted as their consultant in the development of these models which have proved invaluable in the teaching workshops.

Practitioners will gain much stimulation and satisfaction from treating patients with such a variety of soft tissue and joint conditions. Patients will benefit from receiving prompt and efficient therapy, thus avoiding the all too common problem within the National Health Service of long waiting lists for hospital appointments.

This book will reinforce the practice and teaching of injecting joints and soft tissue disorders or lesions, thus achieving the aim of imparting the ability to 'inject with confidence'.

Trevor Silver
January 1996

PREFACE TO SECOND EDITION

I have conducted many practical skills workshops teaching joint and soft tissue injection techniques. More than 5000 doctors have attended these sessions conducted in the United Kingdom and throughout Europe, Asia and Africa. Interestingly, it is not just the minor surgery list in the NHS that has encouraged this increased learning activity, as family practitioners worldwide are becoming much more interested in developing their skills and providing expert joint injection services to their patients. This updated and revised edition includes most of the injection skills family practitioners would want to undertake in their daily practice, and provides most of the answers to questions raised by doctors wishing to provide this service to their patients.

Trevor Silver
September 1998

PREFACE TO THIRD EDITION

This manual provides detailed instruction regarding steroid injection of joint and soft tissue lesions. The evidence base for these therapies is still sparse and has not advanced since the second edition was published. In spite of this, the consensus of opinion appears to support the value of this form of therapy and general practitioners, rheumatologists and orthopaedic surgeons continue to rely on these techniques and principles of therapy. Increasing numbers of GPs worldwide are attending lectures and practical skills workshops, either to learn or to refresh their knowledge of and skills in joint injection therapies.

This third edition benefits from an additional chapter by Dr David Silver, Consultant Radiologist, who has a special interest in musculoskeletal imaging. He elucidates the role of the hospital specialist in the further management of these disorders. Particular attention is paid to those patients who do not respond to initial injection therapy and where specialist referral may be advisable. The need for imaging, particularly the use of ultrasound, magnetic resonance imaging and image-guided intervention is discussed.

It is my expectation that as this subject is practised by increasing numbers of practitioners, more evidence will be forthcoming. The need to agree criteria for diagnosis, techniques of injection and therapy will inevitably facilitate the organisation of more meaningful and informative studies.

More research is needed to establish a uniform method for defining these individual disorders and standardising injection techniques, as well as developing outcome measures that are valid, reliable and responsive in these study populations.

Trevor Silver
September 2001

PREFACE TO FOURTH EDITION

The fact that the publishers have requested a fourth edition of this book confirms that interest in injecting joints and soft tissues continues to flourish.

General practitioners and hospital doctors not only in the UK, but worldwide, are finding that these practical skills are rewarding in primary care as well as in hospital care. The fact that this book is now published in several languages confirms this interest.

Since writing the last edition there has been a noticeable increase in published work, trials and reviews of the literature on the whole range of treatments used in musculoskeletal conditions. Thus, the evidence base is now very comprehensive and a recent restricted Medline search produced over 3500 references. Consequently 'injecting with confidence' is not just a matter of learning about the presentation of the many conditions responding to this form of therapy. Rather, it is the added confidence produced by this evidence base that this subject is now accepted both clinically and therapeutically.

Viscosupplementation is increasingly used to treat a variety of joints with the added prospects of success and prolongation of pain relief. This edition includes recent references and I would encourage readers to read the relevant papers to broaden their horizons of knowledge and so expand their confidence in their management of these conditions.

The evidence for the success of teaching and practical skills workshops, recently published, further confirms my confidence that this subject is now on a much more substantial foundation educationally. It is rewarding to realise that my experience of the last 15 years or so in teaching this subject with practical skills workshops, using simulator models and lectures, has been rewarded by the increasing evidence of a larger number of doctors continuing to practise these skills.

Trevor Silver
February 2007

PREFACE TO FIFTH EDITION

The popularity of this book has been further enhanced by the increasing interest of professionals treating musculoskeletal disorders. Physiotherapists and sports medicine specialists and podiatrists are increasingly combining steroid injections with physiotherapeutic measures of treatment. Because of this, it is necessary that information is available to all practitioners so that a comprehensive approach to successful therapy is achieved.

I am delighted to welcome David MacLellan as a contributing author. His contribution as a sports medicine specialist and physiotherapist complements this book.

General practitioners worldwide are increasingly injecting corticosteroids and this book contributes to their education, as well as their continuing need to attend practical skills workshops and courses.

This edition has further included sections on the elbow joint and iliotibial band syndrome. Further updating on the concepts of greater trochanter pain syndrome is included.

Our aim is to ensure that all therapists have a comprehensive and clear handbook that ensures a high standard of success in treating these conditions.

The increase, worldwide of physical exercise and recreation as the key to good health and longevity makes this book an essential tool towards the education of the many general practitioners, physiotherapists, orthopaedic physicians, surgeons, podiatrists and radiologists. It is interesting that so many disciplines are increasingly engaging in treating these musculoskeletal disorders.

Trevor Silver
October 2010

INTRODUCTION

Injecting with confidence

The development of relatively insoluble corticosteroids has provided doctors with a most useful and effective treatment for the painful musculoskeletal lesions that commonly occur in soft tissues and inflammatory arthropathies. Corticosteroids are potent anti-inflammatory and anti-allergic compounds presented in injectable form in sterile-packed ampoules and vials.

Patients present to their general practitioners (GPs) as a first contact, complaining of pain caused by soft tissue lesions affecting tendons, tendon sheaths or tenoperiosteal junctions, or of painful joints themselves. The cause of these problems is often repetitive strain of a tendon, sport or occupationally induced, resulting in tenderness and pain on movement of the affected structure. Although many of these conditions may be self-limiting, effective treatment using steroid injections is often dramatic and, when accurately diagnosed and skilfully injected, produces relief in most cases.

Both hospital doctors and GPs are ideally placed to treat these disorders, and as most of these patients present in the primary care setting, these problems, quite properly, are considered to be an important part of the general practice curriculum.

Knowledge of the functional (clinical) anatomy, together with learning each individual skill or technique of injection, leads to confidence in treating all these disorders, and it is the aim of this book to provide a comprehensive knowledge and demonstration of skills in an illustrative way, thus imparting to every practitioner the ability to 'inject with confidence'. Making an accurate anatomical diagnosis implies a specific indication for treatment by steroid injection, thus assuring the patient prompt relief. There is no place nowadays for treatment by trial and error. For example, the practitioner who sees a patient with shoulder pain and injects steroid before making an anatomical diagnosis, arranging then to review in one to two weeks' time in the hope of providing relief, is not acceptable. Rather, the doctor should always be in the position of reassuring the patient of prompt relief of pain and of having made an accurate diagnosis before giving treatment.

Practitioners will complement injection therapy as appropriate with analgesic drugs and physiotherapy. They will also be able to advise rest of the affected part for 24–48 hours after the injection and suitable mobilisation thereafter, leading to a resumption of full activity.

I INCIDENCE

I INCIDENCE

There are over eight million people in the UK who are suffering from some form of rheumatic disease and it has been estimated that about one-fifth of all general practitioner (GP) consultations may be attributed to some form of rheumatological or musculoskeletal problem.

Shoulder complaints account for one in every 170 adult patient consultations per year, whereas back problems may account for one in 30 adult patient consultations annually. Thus it is apparent that back problems are approximately five times more common in practice than are shoulder problems.[1] Even so, GPs may well expect to see 20–30 shoulder problems a year in a practice of average list size. Billings and Mole recorded in a prospective study in a London general practice that 10.6% of patients presented with a new rheumatological problem.[2] Of these, 30% were lumbosacral problems, 15% cervical spine problems, 26% degenerative joint disease and 20% soft tissue non-articular rheumatism. Trauma, including sports injuries, accounted for 35% of these problems. The incidence in English and Dutch general practice has been estimated at 6.6–25 per 1000 registered patients per year.[3] The lower annual reported incidence occurred in England and Wales and the higher figure in The Netherlands. In assessing the frequency of the cause of shoulder pain, glenohumeral instability is more likely in under-25 year olds, tendinitis ('impingement') in the 25–40-year age group and frozen shoulder (adhesive capsulitis) in the over-40-year-old age group, with a higher incidence in individuals with diabetes. The term 'impingement' means that the inflamed supraspinatus tendon impinges under the acromion process. Inflammatory joint disease accounts for about 5.5% of these problems, and there is often a case for injecting an inflamed joint with steroid, providing a clinical diagnosis of the type of arthritis has been confirmed beforehand.

It is therefore immediately apparent that GPs are well placed to diagnose and effectively treat all these disorders in their own surgeries, if for no other reason than that the patient will then be assured of prompt and effective treatment for what is often a painful and disabling condition, thus eliminating the frequent long delay many patients experience in obtaining hospital outpatient clinic appointments.

Confirming a diagnosis of these conditions involves examining the active, passive and resisted movements of muscles and affected joints, and relating these to the clinical anatomy. Where there is doubt, X-rays, blood investigations, including erythrocyte sedimentation rate, magnetic resonance imaging and ultrasound scan, may all be helpful in differential diagnosis. A careful history, including the onset of pain, trauma, occupational hazards, sports, gardening and housework, is essential. This careful assessment will give the practitioner confidence in managing these lesions accurately and successfully.

Evidence base

Evidence for the effectiveness of therapy using steroid injections in soft tissue lesions is largely inconclusive. Many studies have been published drawing attention to treatment with intra-articular steroids, physiotherapy or non-steroidal anti-inflammatory drugs. Three systematic reviews were published in 1995, 1996 and 1997.[4-6]

Much of the evidence for the effectiveness of steroids and physiotherapy has been anecdotal. Many of the clinical trials published have demonstrated low patient numbers, a lack of agreed diagnostic criteria and a lack of uniformity in the injection techniques. This has inevitably led to polarised camps of opinion regarding soft tissue lesion and joint injection therapies

It is accepted that the most common lesions causing shoulder pain are those of the rotator cuff and pericapsulitis (frozen shoulder). Moreover, in injecting rotator cuff and frozen shoulder lesions it must be noted that the lesion is in the soft tissue of the rotator cuff tendons, each of which blends with the capsule of the shoulder joint. Consequently, it is not necessary to inject steroid into the glenohumeral joint space but rather to bathe the inflamed tendinitis lesions that lie in the joint capsule itself with steroid solution, with the effect of reducing the inflammation.

Discussion regarding the accurate placement of intra-articular steroids has drawn attention to the fact that steroids should be injected into the synovial joint space to ensure effectiveness in treating arthropathies.[7] It must be emphasised that the success in treating all soft tissue lesions, and especially those affecting the shoulder, is accurate anatomical diagnosis. Rotator cuff lesions require steroid placement within the capsule of the shoulder joint. Tendinitis lesions, e.g. bicipital tendinitis, require injection into the synovial sheath. Arthropathies, e.g. osteoarthritis of the acromioclavicular joint, require placement of the steroid in the joint space.

Again, many of the published studies have involved patients treated in a hospital setting, although the majority of patients with shoulder disorders are treated in the primary care setting. More information is available on the incidence and prognosis of shoulder disorders in primary care since the few epidemiological studies conducted in general practice in Holland (Leiden in 1994 and Amsterdam in 1993).

The aim of treatment is always to resolve pain and improve mobility and function. Conclusive evidence is not available from the published studies of long-term benefit from steroid injection therapy because of the poor quality of methods. There is more evidence of short-term efficacy, particularly for triamcinolone injections. Also, a history of strain or overuse and a short duration of symptoms before presentation to the doctor were shown in one study to predict a speedy recovery in patients.[8]

A study by van der Windt *et al* demonstrated that short-term benefits of steroid injection on capsulitis were superior to those of physiotherapy, with 77% of patients reporting complete recovery or much improvement after steroid injection therapy.[9] Another published randomised trial conducted in primary care reported significant differences in the effects of steroid injection and physiotherapy on shoulder disorders;[10] it reported a 75% success rate after five weeks of treatment with steroid injection compared with 20% for physiotherapy.

Therefore, although more carefully controlled trials of therapy for soft tissue disorders are needed, in recent years there has been an increasing interest in using steroid injection therapy. Since 1990 the author has conducted an increasing number of teaching workshops in diagnosis and injection methods, mainly for GPs and hospital doctors in training. It may be that, in the NHS in the UK, the introduction of minor surgery list procedures, which include joint injection, has encouraged more GPs to learn these skills. This interest has certainly increased in Europe and further afield where GPs are enthusiastic to learn these skills.

Since writing the fourth edition of this book there has been a demonstrable increase in the publication of evidence to support the use of steroid injections in joint and soft tissue disorders. There has also been useful evidence that supports the teaching of injection techniques in the practice of physical medicine and rehabilitation as well as the implementation of objective assessment to measure the attainment of these skills.[11-14]

Further controlled trials of triamcinolone injection, singly or combined with physiotherapy, for shoulder adhesive capsulitis have shown that injection improves shoulder-related disability, and physiotherapy improves the range of movement.[15] A meta-analysis review of 26 references in 2005 concluded that subacromial corticosteroid injections are effective for improvement of rotator cuff tendinitis and that they were more effective than non-steroidal anti-inflammatory drug (NSAID) medication, and that higher doses may be better than lower doses for subacromial injection.[16] Two primary care trials of treatment for shoulder disorders suggested no long-term differences in outcome between patients with shoulder pain treated with different clinical interventions in different clinical settings or having different clinical diagnoses. Baseline clinical characteristics of this consulting population, rather than the randomised treatments they received, were the most powerful predictors of outcome.[17] A survey of GPs in 2005, to determine the type of joint and soft tissue injections carried out by GPs (360), concluded that most carry out some joint and soft tissue injections, but that these are limited to knees, shoulders and elbows. Many GPs find it hard to maintain their skills and confidence. Training targeted at this group, based in practices and using (simulator) models, is likely to increase the number of patients receiving timely injections in general practice.[18]

General principles

As in everything in medicine, it is always wise to take a very careful and complete history – so often the clinician makes a diagnosis before even examining the patient. For example, it is well known that tendon rupture may be hereditary, and a careful history may well reveal that a patient with an Achilles or a long head of biceps tendon problem also had a mother or grandmother with a similar problem. Naturally this would alert one to the fact that it would be unwise to inject steroid around that tendon. Steroids are harmful substances when used inappropriately and, in the present climate of litigation, should never be injected into the substance of a tendon. A patient suffering a tendon rupture who has had a steroid injection in the one to two weeks beforehand would all too often be advised that this was because he or she had received a steroid injection, but in actual fact the situation would be likely to have been related to the hereditary nature of the condition. It is wise to make an accurate anatomical diagnosis on each patient, by careful examination and demonstration of the functional anatomy. This is particularly important when diagnosing the cause of shoulder pain. A good understanding of the anatomy of the shoulder joint, its capsule and the rotator cuff will enable a diagnosis of the condition that the doctor knows will specifically respond to treatment with a steroid injection. This applies to all the conditions that may so easily be treated in the GP surgery, and these will be described in detail in the following chapters.

An aseptic technique should be used for every injection. Steroids are potent anti-inflammatories and in the presence of infection can spell disaster. Consequently, in the presence of local sepsis, such as cellulitis, furunculosis or other staphylococcal infection, introducing a steroid by injection should be avoided. Similarly, any suspicion of sepsis in the joint is an absolute contraindication to injecting steroids. In the presence of systemic infections, one must also exercise caution when using steroids. In the early days when tuberculosis was prevalent, clinicians exercised great caution and avoided the use of steroid medication for fear of exacerbating the illness, and this warning must still be valid today. In fact, in some areas, an increased incidence of tuberculosis is again evident, and vigilance is advised.

The defence organisations advise their members to wear sterile gloves when undertaking minor surgery procedures, including joint injections. Always be seen to wash the hands beforehand, and where possible use a 'no-touch' aseptic technique.

Always use single-dose vials or ampoules where possible, to avoid introducing contaminants into the injection solutions.

Sterilise the injection area and the vial cap using 70% alcohol (surgical spirit). This is cheap to purchase and may be obtained in bulk. This allows the operator to swab liberally and ensures safe working conditions. Nowadays most doctors have ready access to gamma-irradiated sterile syringes and needles, which may only be used once and then safely disposed of.

Inject carefully and unhurriedly. This is mentioned deliberately in order to underline that the patient may often be apprehensive before what is reputedly a painful injection. It is necessary to cast an appearance of calm in the operator and so help towards making the patient more relaxed. A relaxed patient will have more relaxed muscles, thus ensuring that the injection allows the solution simply to glide in, making the whole procedure easy and requiring no visible force on the syringe plunger. In fact with all these injections the agent should be felt to glide in easily and require the minimum of force to introduce. As in all procedures, there is the exception, and it must be stated that when injecting the denser fibrous tissues of tenoperiosteal junctions, as in tennis and golfer's elbow (lateral and medial epicondylitis), there may well be some resistance to the injection; in these cases it is wise to ensure that the needle is firmly secured to the syringe.

Frequency of injection

There is no firm rule regarding how frequently one may inject one lesion or one person with several lesions. Generally one must assume that the lowest number of injections and the lowest dose practicable should be employed. Although intra-articular steroid preparations are not likely to be systemically absorbed, some absorption will inevitably take place.

Consequently, the more frequently injections are given, the greater the likelihood, hypothetically, that the patient may exhibit all the unattractive qualities of long-term steroid administration, and we are all aware of the undesirable effects that this produces. One only needs to remember the patients who in the past were prescribed long-term steroids for asthma or rheumatoid arthritis to recall the possible side-effects.

The general advice usually proffered is that, where necessary, one may inject a steroid at no more than three- to four-weekly intervals, and probably no more than three or four times into one lesion in the course of any one year. The author's view is that if two or three injections have not produced the desired and expected benefit, one should review the diagnosis. Certainly, if added steroid medication is given, one should expect the patient to experience the undesirable effects associated with prolonged steroid medication.

Choice of steroid

There are many steroid preparations on the market for intra-articular and soft tissue use. They are relatively insoluble, consequently exerting a longer-lasting local effect, and are not absorbed systemically to any great degree. They should be injected into the substance of the lesion, the tender spot or the joint space. In some lesions it is advisable to mix the steroid beforehand with local anaesthetic, whereas in others such mixing will not take place; this will be discussed when describing each individual technique. Some preparations are marketed with steroid and local anaesthetic pre-mixed. This has the disadvantage of not allowing the operator the flexibility of titrating the preferred amounts or doses of local anaesthetic or steroid for each particular injection. This may be quite important when, for example, treating a painful recurrent condition, such as plantar fasciitis, and the requirement for local anaesthetic may vary in type and quantity (see following page).

Three commonly used preparations are:

- hydrocortisone acetate 25 mg/ml (Hydrocortistab®)
- methylprednisolone acetate 40 mg/ml (Depo-Medrone®)
- triamcinolone hexacetonide 20 mg/ml (Aristospan®)*
- triamcinolone acetonide 40 mg/ml (Kenalog®).

These preparations increase in potency and length of action in the order of the list, and conversely they decrease in volume for dose in that order. This means in effect that triamcinolone acetonide will produce a longer-lasting effect in a comparatively smaller volume dose. This effect is beneficial clinically if one recalls that some of these injections, for example those into dense tissue such as the tenoperiosteal junction in tennis elbow, can be quite painful. Therefore, the smaller the injection volume the better, to decrease the pain of the injection while at the same time delivering a very effective dose of steroid.

There are some occasions on which one will wish to mix the steroid with local anaesthetic, and others when it is inadvisable to add local anaesthetic; these will be discussed in the ensuing technique descriptions. Both hydrocortisone acetate and triamcinolone acetonide have product licences allowing one to pre-mix with lidocaine or bupivacaine. Methylprednisolone does not have such a licence, but the manufacturer of Depo-Medrone® produces a ready-mixed preparation with lidocaine 10 mg/ml.

---

*In the past 2 years production of Lederspan® ceased. Triamcinolone hexacetonide is only available as Aristospan® 20 mg/ml made by Harvard Pilgrim Health Care (USA).

Contraindications to the use of steroids

Active tuberculosis, ocular herpes and acute psychosis are considered to be absolute contraindications to glucocorticoid therapy, although the minimal systemic activity after local injection may permit its cautious use. Never inject steroids into infected joints. Where there is any suspicion, always aspirate any effusion and send it to the laboratory for culture of micro-organisms before considering injecting. Similarly, diabetes, hypertension, osteoporosis and hyperthyroidism are listed as possible contraindications. Don't inject steroid into a joint with a prosthesis. Hypersensitivity to one of the ingredients of the injection is a definite contraindication. In pregnancy one should take care; corticosteroids are certainly contraindicated in the first 16 weeks of pregnancy. However, it may be a fine clinical judgement whether or not to use steroids, for example in carpal tunnel syndrome, which is a common condition in middle pregnancy; caution must undoubtedly be exercised. It must also be remembered that prolonged or repeated use in weight-bearing joints may result in further degeneration. No more than two or three joints in a patient should be treated at the same time.

Never attempt to inject into the substance of a tendon, but always ensure that the steroid is injected into the space between the tendon and the tendon sheath in tenosynovitis.

Local anaesthetic

There are occasions on which one will wish to use local anaesthetic mixed with the steroid, and others when this is not advised. Lidocaine plain 1% is probably the most effective and commonly used agent. This anaesthetic is extremely effective; its onset is immediate and its effect will last for two to four hours. Where it is desirable to produce a longer-lasting local anaesthetic effect, for example in the case of a recurrent plantar fasciitis which is a very painful condition, it is sometimes useful to use bupivacaine plain 0.25% or 0.5% (Marcain® plain). The effect of this may last from five to 16 hours.

With both these local agents, it is undesirable and unnecessary to use adrenaline mixed with the anaesthetic solution.

Post-injection advice

Following a steroid injection the patient is well advised to rest the joint or affected part for two or three days. Patients are advised not to carry heavy bags or shopping for a couple of days. Also the patient should not undertake any of the painful movements for a couple of days, after which a slow return to normal pain-free activity is permissible. Occasionally the use of a sling following injection of a painful shoulder or tennis elbow is acceptable, but this should be discarded after the pain has resolved.

References

1 Department of Health and Social Services (1986) *Morbidity Statistics from General Practice: the third national study (1981–82)*. HMSO, London.

2 Billings RA and Mole KF (1977) Rheumatology in general practice: a survey in world rheumatology tear, 1977. *J R Coll Gen Pract.* **27**: 721–5.

3 Croft P (1993) Soft tissue rheumatism. In: AJ Silman and MC Hochberg (eds) *Epidemiology of the Rheumatic Diseases*. Oxford Medical Publications, Oxford.

4 Van der Windt DA *et al* (1995) The efficacy of NSAIDs for shoulder complaints. *J Clin Epidemiol.* **48**: 691–704.

5 Van der Heijden GJ *et al* (1996) Steroid injection for shoulder disorders: a systematic review of randomised clinical trails. *Br J Gen Pract.* **46**: 309–16.

6 Van der Heijden GJ *et al* (1997) Physiotherapy for patients with soft tissue shoulder disorders: a systematic review of randomised clinical trials. *BMJ.* **315**: 25–30.

7 Jones A *et al* (1993) Importance of placement of intra-articular steroid injections. *BMJ.* **307**: 1329–30.

8 Chard M *et al* (1988) The long-term outcome of rotator cuff tendinitis: a review study. *Br J Rheumatol.* **27**: 385–9.

9 Van der Windt DA *et al* (1997) *Steroid Injection or Physiotherapy for Capsulitis of the Shoulder: a randomised clinical trial in primary care*. Privately published.

10 Winters JC *et al* (1997) Comparison of physiotherapy, manipulation and steroid injection for treating shoulder complaints in general practice: a randomised single blind study. *BMJ.* **314**: 1320–5.

11 Cucurullo S *et al* (2004) Musculoskeletal injection skills competency: a method for development and assessment. *Am J Phys Med Rehabil.* **83**(6): 479–84.

12 Grahame R (2005) *Efficacy of 'Hands On' Soft Tissue Injection Courses for General Practitioners using Live Patients*. Poster presentation at Rheumatology conference. Personal communication.

13 Kneebone R (2004) *Teaching and Learning Basic Skills using Multimedia and Models*. PhD Thesis.

14 Bell AD and Conaway D (2005) Corticosteroid injections for painful shoulders. *Int J Clin Pract*. **59**: 1178–86.

15 Ryans I *et al* (2005) A randomised controlled trial of intra-articular triamcinolone and/or physiotherapy in shoulder capsulitis. *Rheumatol*. **44**: 529–35.

16 Arroll B and Goodyear-Smith F (2005) Corticosteroid injections for painful shoulder: a meta-analysis. *Br J Gen Pract*. **55**: 224–8.

17 Thomas E *et al* (2005) Two pragmatic trials of treatment for shoulder disorders in primary care: generalisability, course and prognostic indicators. *Ann Rheum Dis*. **64**: 1056–61.

18 Liddell WG *et al* (2005) Joint and soft tissue injections: a survey of general practitioners. *Rheumatol*. **44**: 1043–6.

2 MEDICO-LEGAL ISSUES

2 MEDICO-LEGAL ISSUES

Because steroids have, over the years, been notable in the number of undesirable side-effects as well as their magical clinical effects, their prescription and use have come under severe scrutiny by the public at large. To this end, the legal professions on both sides of the Atlantic have enjoyed a bonanza of medical litigation, much of which has been spurious. Nevertheless, media attention has been prolific, and words of caution to the medical profession will not be untoward in this manual.

Steroids are potent anti-inflammatory drugs, but at the same time inappropriate or over use may well spell disaster for a patient. There are several concepts that should be considered, which should be incorporated into the practising physician's normal daily routine.

Pain after injection

These injection procedures are often painful at the time of injection, and many will give rise to pain after the local anaesthetic effect has worn off, sometimes for up to 48 hours after the injection. It is therefore wise to warn every patient of this possibility, as forewarned is forearmed. Simple advice should be given to take appropriate analgesic tablets: 2 × 500 mg paracetamol tablets four-hourly as required while the pain lasts.

More importantly, the development of pain increasing in severity some 48 hours after injection may herald the very serious complication of a septic arthritis. Warning the patient of this very rare complication is wise, and informing him to return immediately to the doctor for reassessment in such an event may well avoid a serious cause for litigation.

Informed consent

A few minutes of explaining the condition, together with the implications of any side-effects, to the patient is time well spent. The fact that many of these conditions are self-limiting makes it all the more important for patients to be allowed to make an informed decision on whether they would or would not like a steroid injection. Naturally, when they are made aware that a frozen shoulder, for example, may take up to three years to get better without treatment and that a steroid injection may provide improvement of the same condition in two weeks, they are well able to make that decision for themselves. I prefer to allow, whenever possible, my patient actively to make the decision of whether or not to have such an injection. That, I believe, is informed consent.

Specific indication

Making an accurate anatomical diagnosis implies a specific indication for injection therapy. As mentioned previously, there is no real place for the clinical trial, as giving a specific injection for a specific condition will always imply correct and accepted treatment. No-one can then complain afterwards that the treatment was inappropriate.

Full records

One cannot emphasise enough the importance of maintaining full, legible, accurate notes of each patient attendance. To include the history, subjective findings, full examination findings, diagnosis and management, together with all the doses and quantities of any prescribed drugs, should be routine. In any subsequent litigation, this will certainly impart the most favourable impression of a competent practitioner.

Technique of the procedure

Demonstrating careful and efficient management in the treatment room creates a good impression. Washing the hands, wearing sterile gloves, using single-dose vials and having clean surroundings are all important. Sterilising the operation site and putting an Elastoplast® plaster over the injection site after the procedure are both evidence of care and go a long way to ensuring that the patient is receiving the best possible attention.

Untoward complications of steroid injection
Lipodystrophy

When steroid is inadvertently injected subcutaneously, lipodystrophy may occur. This will result in dimpling of the skin, which may well upset a patient, especially if they have not been warned beforehand. Because these lesions are quite superficial, this effect occurs more commonly after injections for tennis and golfer's elbow. Although the more potent steroids have the reputation of being susceptible in this respect, and it is wise to warn patients of this possibility, I believe any subcutaneous injection of steroid may cause lipodystrophy.

Loss of skin pigment

Injecting steroid subcutaneously in patients with dark skin may occasionally leave a small area of pigment loss. Again it is wise to warn of this possibility and pre-empt any cause for subsequent complaint.

Repeat injections at the same site are not recommended. There have been cases of tendon rupture, for example of the patellar tendon following repeated injection of the infrapatellar bursa of the knee joint, and practitioners should be aware of this complication.

Other tendons known to rupture are the Achilles, of which mention has already been made, the bicipital (long head of biceps), which is known to rupture spontaneously, and the palmar flexor tendons. In all of these cases, caution is advised in the use of steroid injection.

A 2005 review (58 references) of injectable steroids in modern practice suggested that corticosteroids of low solubility are thought to have the longest duration of action. Intra-articular steroids have been shown to be safe and effective for repeated use (every three months) for up to two years, with no detectable joint space narrowing being seen. The accuracy of injections affects their outcomes. Post-injection flare, facial flushing and skin and fat atrophy are the most common side-effects. Systemic complications of injectable steroids are rare.[1]

However, a disturbing report of fatal necrotising fasciitis following therapeutic injection of a shoulder joint was published in 2005. Although this is the only reference I have discovered in a Medline search for the past 15 years, it remains a salutary reminder of the need for maximum care and sterility whenever undertaking this work.[2]

References

1   Cole B *et al* (2005) Injectable corticosteroids in modern practice. *J Am Acad Orthop Surg.* **13**(1): 37–46.

2   Unglaub F *et al* (2005) Necrotizing fasciitis following therapeutic injection in a shoulder joint [in German]. *Orthopade.* **34**(3): 250–2.

3 THE SHOULDER

3 THE SHOULDER

There are many causes of pain in or around the shoulder joint. It is important to be accurate in their diagnosis, to determine those that will respond well to treatment with steroid injection into the site of the lesion or the joint itself. These are:

- rotator cuff tendinitis (subscapularis, infraspinatus)
- supraspinatus tendinitis (may be calcific)
- frozen shoulder (adhesive capsulitis)
- subacromial bursitis
- bicipital tendinitis (long head of the biceps)
- osteoarthritis of the acromioclavicular joint
- acute arthropathies, e.g. rheumatoid, psoriasis and other seronegative arthropathies.

Presentation and diagnosis

Shoulder pain occurs most commonly in the middle-aged or older age group of patients, and the incidence appears to plateau at about 45 years of age. Women are affected more frequently than men.

Most 'painful shoulder' conditions that present in general practice are caused by soft tissue lesions affecting the rotator cuff. These painful lesions occur in tendons or tenoperiosteal junctions. They are naturally tender on palpation, or create pain on active or resisted movements of the affected part. Osteoarthritis and inflammatory arthritis are less common causes. Osteoarthritis practically never affects the shoulder joint but commonly affects the acromioclavicular joint in patients who are over 50 years old.

Lesions of any or all the tendons of the rotator cuff may be caused by repetitive or acute occupational strain. Acute strain of the supraspinatus tendon occurs most commonly in sports injuries or gardening activities. Bicipital tendinitis, a form of tenosynovitis affecting the tendon sheath of the long head of the biceps, similarly follows sports or tree-lopping activity. It should be specifically diagnosed when it occurs, as the treatment involves injecting steroid, mixed with local anaesthetic, directly into the tendon sheath to achieve immediate relief. Frozen shoulder is the most chronic of shoulder conditions and indicates strain of all the rotator cuff tendons, causing a capsulitis. The earlier this condition is treated, the less likely it is to become chronic. Conditions leading to immobilisation, such as strokes and coronary thrombosis, often results in the shoulder–arm syndrome, owing to a reflex sympathetic dystrophy. Fortunately, present-day therapy of these conditions tends to lead to earlier mobilisation, and consequently shoulder–arm syndromes have become quite rare.

Impingement syndrome is a diagnosis that has become fashionable in the past few years. It is characterised by pain at the lateral tip of the shoulder, on abduction of the arm, and is actually supraspinatus tendinitis. It is due to swelling and inflammation of the supraspinatus muscle impinging under the lateral tip of the acromion as the arm is actively abducted. The condition may be likely where there has been previous trauma to the lateral tip of the acromion. Injection of corticosteroid is still the treatment of choice in the first instance, and provides significant improvements in shoulder function with regard to range of movement, strength and disturbance of sleep.[1]

Pitfalls in diagnosis

Referred pain to the tip of the shoulder

Patients may complain of pain in the shoulder, which may be referred to the C5 dermatome by other conditions. These produce pain that is not necessarily related to muscle or tendon movement, for example:

- bronchogenic carcinoma of the apex of the lung (Pancoast tumour)
- cervical spine disc lesions or nerve entrapments
- heart problems
- diaphragmatic problems
- oesophageal conditions.

A high index of clinical suspicion is necessary to recognise a Pancoast tumour. This bronchogenic carcinoma affecting the apex of the lung may well produce pain referred to the tip of the shoulder. It is a great advantage in conditions such as these if the primary contact physician makes an early diagnosis. Where this does not happen, the patient with shoulder pain who is referred to a hospital rheumatological clinic may well wait up to three or four months for an outpatient appointment, by which time a late diagnosis of bronchogenic carcinoma can be catastrophic for the patient. In such instances, there is a strong case for general practitioners (GPs) who see their patients often at the onset of symptoms to be expert at diagnosing and treating these soft tissue disorders.

Polymyalgia rheumatica is another condition that presents early in the general practice setting. Doctors are only too well aware of the classical history of severe pain and stiffness affecting the hips and proximal thighs, together with the shoulders and upper arms, early in the morning. Occasionally the onset may affect one shoulder only at the start of the disease, leading to some difficulty in differential diagnosis. What better achievement for the practitioner who diagnoses this condition at such an early stage? Being well aware of the presentation of all these disorders enhances the doctor's skill in diagnosis and early effective therapy. In this example, a simple erythrocyte sedimentation rate (ESR) blood test may be all that is necessary to confirm the diagnosis of polymyalgia.

In diabetes, frozen shoulder occurs more frequently, and occasionally finding a patient whose condition has been slow to respond to steroid injection should alert one to this diagnosis, especially in a female aged over 50 years.

A good rule is to test the urine for sugar in a patient, more usually female, whose frozen shoulder problem has failed to improve with two or three steroid injections.

Pain referred to the deltoid insertion

Pain referred to the deltoid insertion halfway down the lateral side of the upper arm may occur in any of the rotator cuff lesions and should not tempt the doctor to inject steroid at this site. The techniques for injection of the shoulder lesions described later in the text are always the ones that should be used.

Functional anatomy

Understanding the functional or clinical anatomy of the shoulder will ensure that a specific diagnosis is made, as well as giving confidence in the skill of accurate injection. Lack of this knowledge has in the past prevented the practitioner from developing the confidence to know that the injecting needle is accurately sited. The aim in injecting the shoulder joint for the rotator cuff lesions is to ensure that the needle enters the capsule of the joint. It is not necessary to attempt to place the needle point in the glenohumeral joint space. The lesions essentially being treated are those of the soft tissues that surround the joint and blend with and strengthen the capsule.

The glenohumeral joint consists of the head of the humerus articulating with the glenoid fossa of the scapula. The shallow joint space is no more than 1.5 inches (3.8 cm) in length. The joint is held together by a rather loosely applied voluminous capsule of fibrous tissue, which is considerably strengthened by the three tendons of the rotator cuff that blend with it anteriorly, posteriorly and superiorly respectively from the subscapularis, the infraspinatus together with teres minor, and the supraspinatus. The long head of biceps tendon arises on the superior glenoid tubercle within the capsule of the joint and becomes covered by its own synovial sheath as it lies superiorly in the capsule and it leaves the joint space through an opening in the capsule, passing over the bicipital groove which lies on the anterolateral surface of the head of the humerus, to join the short head of the biceps muscle anteriorly over the upper arm.

The subscapularis lies anteriorly, and internally (medially) rotates the arm; the infraspinatus (lies posteriorly) and teres minor together externally (laterally) rotate and the supraspinatus (lies superiorly) abducts the arm to 90 degrees ('the painful arc').

Because these tendons blend with the capsule of the shoulder joint, it is only necessary to inject into the space enclosed by the joint capsule in order to bathe the inflamed soft tissue lesions in steroid and lidocaine, which effect resolution of the inflammation. Contrary to popular belief it is not necessary to inject into the glenohumeral joint space itself.

The acromioclavicular joint

This is a small plane joint or syntosis where the lateral end of the clavicle articulates with the acromion process of the scapula. The capsular ligament is strengthened by the acromioclavicular ligament. There is a very small joint space that will admit 0.2–0.5 ml of injection fluid.

It must be noted that bicipital tendinitis, which is a tenosynovitis of the sheath of this tendon, and osteoarthritis of the acromioclavicular joint, both common causes of shoulder pain, must be injected as described later for each particular condition. Failure to accurately diagnose and treat these disorders specifically contributes to the lack of success in shoulder injection to which some commentators refer.

Examination of the shoulder

Understanding the above allows a simple routine examination of the shoulder joint, which will accurately determine the source of the pain.

First assess the cervical spine for the normal range of movements and to ascertain that no pain is referred from the neck to the shoulder. With the patient standing up, check:

- forward flexion – ask the patient to bend the head forward as far as possible
- backward flexion – bend the head backwards as far as possible
- head rotation – rotate the head fully to right and then left, and (subjectively) measure any deficit in degrees
- lateral flexion – side bending to right and left sides.

Note any restrictions to these movements and whether any of these movements cause pain in the affected shoulder.

With the patient stripped to the waist, inspect both shoulders to exclude any joint swellings, effusion, signs of arthritis and subacromial bursitis. Test for local points of tenderness. Tenderness of the shoulder over the bicipital tendon lying in the bicipital groove may suggest bicipital tendinitis, whereas tenderness palpated over the lateral tip of the shoulder may alert the examiner to the possibility of supraspinatus tendinitis.

Next examine the full range of active movements. With the patient standing, ask him to do the following:

- abduct both arms to 90 degrees with the palms facing the ceiling. This movement is performed by the supraspinatus. (The 'painful arc' is a term first described by James Cyriax as meaning pain in shoulder on active abduction of the arm). Restriction = supraspinatus tendinitis
- next place both hands on the back of the head (the occiput). This is external rotation and is performed by the infraspinatus. Restriction = infraspinatus tendinitis
- now bring both arms behind the chest and raise the thumbs as high as possible. This movement is internal rotation and is performed by the subscapularis. Restriction = subscapularis tendinitis.

Note any pain or restriction of any of these rotator cuff movements. If all these movements are painful or restricted, the diagnosis of frozen shoulder is implied.

Note the pain caused by any of the specific movements that are reproduced on testing the resisted movements, which will indicate the tendon involved.

Passive movement of the shoulder with one hand placed over the joint may reveal the crepitus present in pericapsulitis (frozen shoulder).

Diagnosis of any lesion is then confirmed by checking the resisted movements. A diagnosis of tendinitis (repetitive strain) may only be confirmed when pain and restricted movement are demonstrated on testing the resisted movements of the tendon.

In the diagnosis of soft tissue lesions always remember to examine the:

1 ACTIVE movements
2 RESISTED movements
3 PASSIVE movements.

What the pain means (see Figure 3.1)

1 Pain on resisted abduction

The patient abducts both arms up to 90 degrees while the examiner applies counterpressure to this movement. If this causes pain, the diagnosis is supraspinatus tendinitis. In this condition, X-ray examination of the shoulder may reveal calcification in the substance of the supraspinatus tendon within the shoulder joint capsule. This is no contraindication to steroid injection, which is very effective. As will be seen, injection of the shoulder is into the capsule, and no attempt is made to inject into the tendon itself.

If pain is experienced when the arms are raised in the range from 90 degrees (horizontal) through to 180 degrees (vertical), this suggests osteoarthritis of the acromioclavicular joint (*see* p. 36).

2 Resisted external rotation

With both elbows pressed into the ribs and with the arms flexed at 90 degrees pointing forwards, the patient pushes the forearms and hands outwards against resistance. Pain indicates infraspinatus tendinitis.

3 Resisted internal rotation

With both elbows tucked into the ribs and both arms flexed at 90 degrees, the patient presses the hands inwards against resistance. Pain indicates subscapularis tendinitis.

4 Resisted supination and flexion of the forearm

The patient flexes the forearms against resistance or supinates the wrist against resistance with the elbow bent to 90 degrees. Pain felt at the tip of the shoulder implies bicipital tendinitis. An alternative test is to resist forward movement of the arm with the elbow extended, producing pain at the tip of the shoulder.

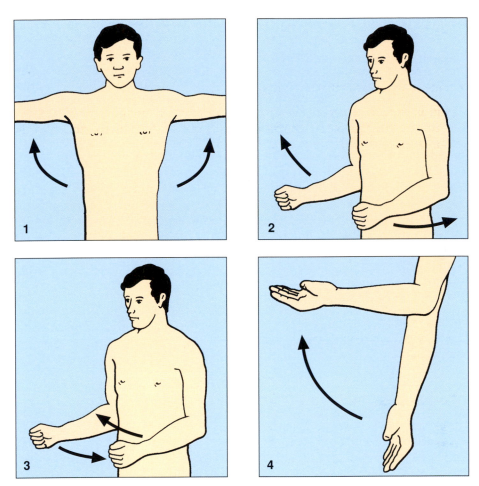

Figure 3.1 What the pain means.

Injection technique

Anterior approach (see Figure 3.2)

The patient sits with the arm loosely at the side and externally rotated. Remember that the aim is to inject into the space within the shoulder joint capsule.

Use a 2 ml syringe with a 1 inch (2.5 cm) needle (blue hub) filled with 1 ml steroid solution mixed with 1 ml lidocaine plain 1%. Advance the needle horizontally and in a slightly lateral direction below the acromion process, lateral to the tip of the coracoid process of the scapula and immediately medial to the head of the humerus, all of which are easily palpated. It is especially simple to palpate the head of the humerus anteriorly while passively rotating the humerus internally and externally with the left hand at the bent elbow. Always inject just medially to the head of the humerus; the needle can then only be in the capsule of the shoulder joint. Inject when no resistance is felt to the plunger. Remember that the steroid is injected into the capsule of the shoulder joint and not into the glenohumeral joint space, which is relatively narrow and small.

After the injection, ask the patient to repeat the active shoulder joint movements. These movements should now be pain-free owing to the use of local anaesthetic which was mixed with the steroid solution.

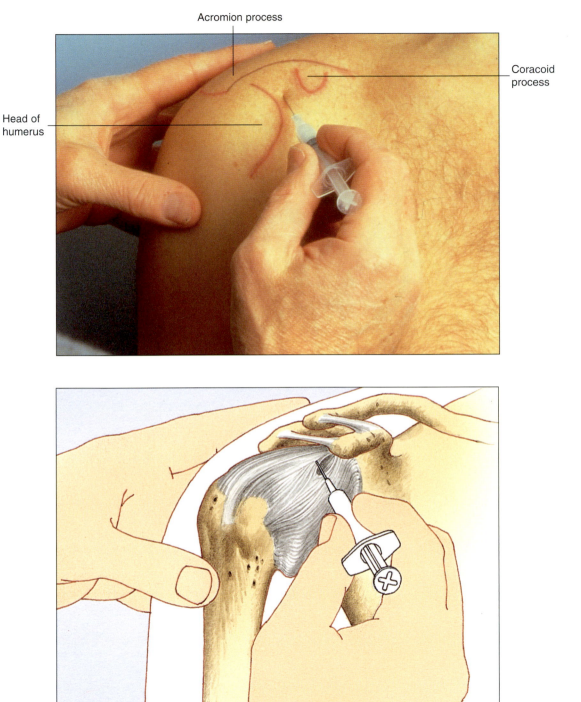

Anterior approach.

Lateral (subacromial) approach (see Figure 3.3)

The patient sits with the arm loosely at the side and not rotated. Palpate the most lateral point of the shoulder and make a thumbnail indentation about 0.5 inch (1.3 cm) below the tip of the acromion process. Use 1 ml steroid mixed with 1 ml lidocaine 1% plain in a 2 ml syringe with a 1.5 inch (3.8 cm) needle. The larger needle is advisable as the subcutaneous fat of the upper arm is often quite thick at this point. Advance the needle medially below the acromion process, horizontally and in a slightly posterior direction along the line of the supraspinous fossa. Inject the solution when 1 inch (2.5 cm) of the needle has been inserted.

In subacromial bursitis there is often an effusion, which feels fluctuant to each side of the acromion process. This may be aspirated before injecting the steroid and local anaesthetic mixture. Subacromial bursitis may occur in gout, in Reiter's syndrome, following trauma or in rheumatoid arthritis. Sometimes it may be caused by hydroxyapatite crystals (99% calcium which forms hydroxyapatite crystals of bone – the mineral of bone). Apart from the presence of an effusion, this condition may be diagnosed by asking the patient to place the arm of the affected side diagonally across the front of the chest. Tapping the point of the elbow will then produce transmitted pain under the acromion process.

In most cases, the shoulder joint communicates with the subacromial space, and apart from aspirating and injecting subacromial bursitis it is useful to use this lateral approach for any of the rotator cuff lesions. Indeed the approach to injecting the shoulder joint is more often a personal choice, as the effect of injecting laterally, anteriorly or posteriorly is the same therapeutically for the rotator cuff and frozen shoulder problems.

Acromion process

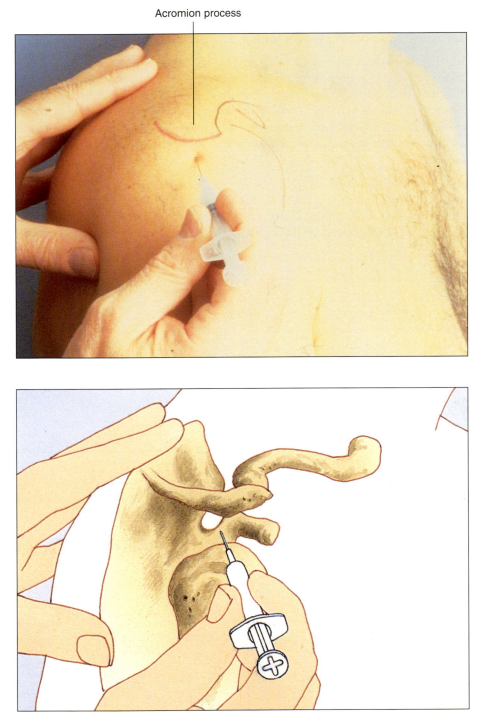

Figure 3.3 Lateral (subacromial) approach.

Posterior approach (see Figure 3.4)

Use 1 ml steroid mixed with 1 ml lidocaine 1% plain in a 2 ml syringe. Use a 1.5 inch (3.8 cm) needle as, again, the subcutaneous fat over the back is quite thick, especially in an obese patient. The patient sits with the back towards the operator. Palpate the posterior tip of the acromion process with the tip of the thumb. Place the index finger of the same hand on the coracoid process. The imaginary line between the index finger and the thumb marks the track of the needle.

Advance the needle from an entry point approximately 1 inch (2.5 cm) below the tip of the thumb (i.e. below the tip of the acromion and medial to the head of the humerus) about 1 inch (2.5 cm) towards the index finger marking the coracoid process. There will be no resistance to the injection, as the needle point will be in the capsule of the shoulder joint.

This approach is suitable for all the rotator cuff lesions and for frozen shoulder.

Acromion process

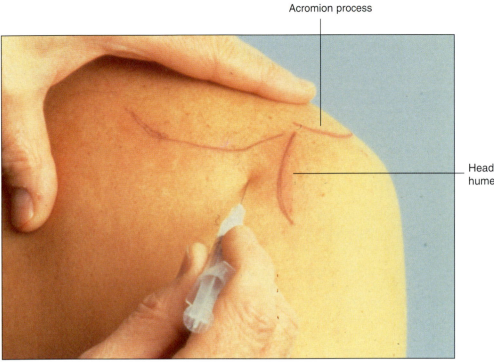

Head of
humerus

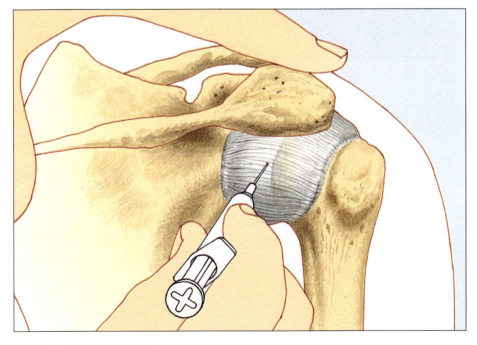

Figure 3.4 Posterior approach.

Bicipital tendinitis

The patient complains of pain over the tip of the shoulder. To distinguish this pain from that due to the rotator cuff tendinitis, examination of the shoulder will reveal:

- tenderness on palpation over the bicipital groove
- pain at the tip of the shoulder on resisted supination (Yergason's test) of the wrist; resisted flexion of the forearm will additionally cause pain over the bicipital groove.

The bicipital groove (the intertubercular sulcus) is palpable at the anterolateral tip of the head of the humerus. When the subject rotates the arm medially and laterally, the groove becomes more easily identifiable.

It must be emphasised that this condition, which is due to strain of the long head of biceps tendon, is in fact a tenosynovitis. To cure this condition, the aim is to inject 1 ml steroid solution mixed with 1 ml lidocaine 1% plain directly into the space between the bicipital tendon and the synovial sheath. Care must be taken not to inject into the substance of the bicipital tendon, which could cause rupture.

Following the injection, if the injection solution is correctly sited the patient will feel immediate relief of the tenderness and the pain felt on resisted supination.

In any form of tendinitis:

1 only diagnose if there is pain on resisted movement
2 pain in the absence of movement may imply other pathology.

Injection technique (see Figure 3.5)

- Use a 2 ml volume syringe with a $\frac{5}{8}$ inch (1.6 cm) needle. Mix 1 ml of steroid with 1 ml lidocaine 1% plain.
- The patient sits with the affected arm loosely by the side but externally rotated. Make a thumbnail indentation directly over the most tender spot in the bicipital groove, which is easily palpated. This is the site of needle entry.
- Inject just below the skin mark, and direct the needle in an upward direction into the bicipital groove. When the needle point enters the substance of the tendon, resistance increases sharply. Maintain gentle pressure on the plunger while at the same time withdrawing the needle slowly until the resistance disappears. At this point the needle is in the synovial sheath, when 2 ml of solution may be injected.

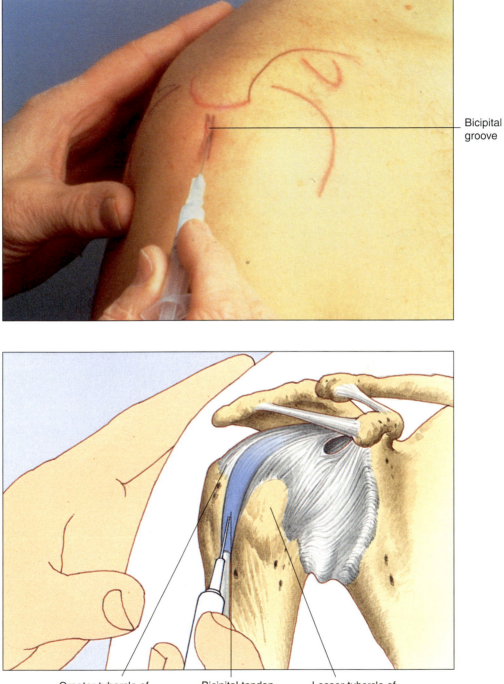

Bicipital
groove

Greater tubercle of
head of humerus

Bicipital tendon
in its sheath

Lesser tubercle of
head of humerus

Figure 3.5 Bicipital tendinitis.

It is rewarding to diagnose and cure this relatively common cause of shoulder pain. In the past, critics of the usage of steroid injection have suggested that many patients with shoulder pain have not always responded to the injection. It is suggested that all too often the clinician has not tested and examined specifically to diagnose bicipital tendinitis, but rather vaguely grouped all shoulder pains to have the more common cause of rotator cuff lesion. Thus, a more complete differential diagnosis will inevitably lead to a higher success rate in the injection treatment of all these shoulder lesions.

Acromioclavicular joint

Osteoarthritis of the acromioclavicular joint is a common cause of pain in the patient aged over 50 years. The patient complains of pain directly over the joint, and the diagnosis is confirmed on examination.

- There may be an osteophyte palpable over the joint space itself, which is an obvious indicator that osteoarthritis is present.
- Abduction of the arm from the horizontal to the vertical position will produce pain over the acromioclavicular joint.
- The arm forcefully adducted across the front of the chest under the chin with the forearm flexed at 90 degrees while protracting the shoulder girdle causes pain over the acromioclavicular joint.
- Forcefully adducting the arm posteriorly across the back of the chest will produce pain at the limit of adduction.

A diagnostic local injection of local anaesthetic will provide relief of pain. Injection of the acromioclavicular joint with corticosteroid does not alter the natural progression of osteoarthritis but is a valuable procedure for longer-term relief.[2]

Injection technique (see Figure 3.6)

The acromioclavicular joint has a very small joint space that will only accept an injection of between 0.2 and 0.5 ml of fluid. Use a 2 ml volume syringe with a $\frac{5}{8}$ inch (1.6 cm) needle. It is not necessary to mix local anaesthetic and inject up to 0.5 ml of triamcinolone acetonide. Carefully palpate the joint space and insert the needle either superiorly with a vertical approach, or anteriorly, ensuring that only the tip of the needle enters the joint space. Although the joint space is sometimes difficult to enter on account of the presence of an osteophyte, it is equally easy to push the needle too far and enter the shoulder capsule from above.

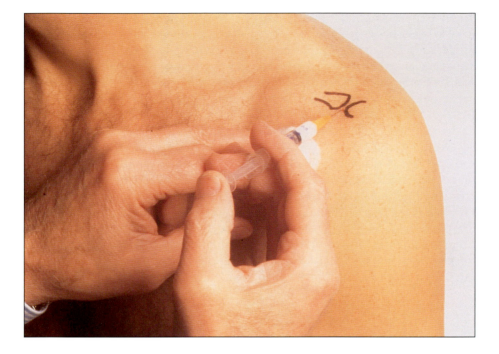

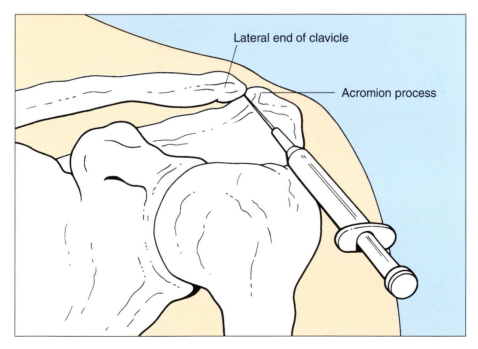

Figure 3.6 Acromioclavicular joint osteoarthritis.

Studies reported in 2005 (a meta-analysis, 26 references) revealed the effectiveness, in terms of symptom improvement, of subacromial corticosteroid injections for rotator cuff tendinitis and frozen shoulder. It was concluded that the effect lasted for nine months and was more effective than non-steroidal anti-inflammatory drugs (NSAIDs) and that higher doses were better than lower doses for subacromial corticosteroid injection.[3] A randomised trial in 2005 reported that the shoulder disability questionnaire score improved in those receiving corticosteroid injection and that physiotherapy improved passive external rotation six weeks after treatment.[4] A cost consequences analysis of local corticosteroid shoulder injection and physiotherapy for new episodes of shoulder pain in primary care reported similar clinical outcomes for both treatment groups, and that corticosteroid injections were the more cost-effective option.[5] A study in 2006 reported that the prevalence of people consulting for shoulder problems in primary care is substantially lower than community-based estimates. Most referrals occur within three months of initial presentation but only a minority are referred to specialists. It is suggested that, in Oxford, GPs may lack confidence in applying precise diagnosis of shoulder conditions.[6]

References

1 Akgun K *et al* (2004) Is local subacromial corticosteroid injection beneficial in subacromial impingement syndrome? *Clin Rheumatol.* **23**(6): 496–500.

2 Buttaci CJ *et al* (2004) Osteoarthritis of the acromioclavicular joint: a review of anatomy, biomechanics, diagnosis and treatment. Review [24 references]. *Am J Phys Med Rehabil.* **83**(10): 791–7.

3 Arroll B and Goodyear-Smith F (2005) Corticosteroid injections for painful shoulder: a meta-analysis. *Br J Gen Pract.* **55**: 224–8.

4 Ryans I *et al* (2005) A randomised controlled trial of intra-articular triamcinolone and/or physiotherapy in shoulder capsulitis. *Rheumatol.* **44**: 529–35.

5 James M *et al* (2005) A cost analysis of local corticosteroid injection and physiotherapy for the treatment of new episodes of unilateral shoulder pain in primary care. *Rheumatol.* **44**(11): 1447–51.

6 Linsell L *et al* (2006) Prevalence and incidence of adults consulting for shoulder conditions in UK primary care: patterns of referral and diagnosis. *Rheumatol.* **45**(2): 215–21.

4 THE WRIST AND HAND

4 THE WRIST AND HAND

Incidence

Soft tissue lesions commonly occur in the wrist joint, hand and fingers. Rheumatoid arthritis and other arthropathies predispose to some of these problems. Osteoarthritis is about four times more common than rheumatoid arthritis. Primary osteoarthritis runs in families as an autosomal dominant trait. The most familiar pattern affects the terminal interphalangeal joints, producing Heberden's nodes, as well as affecting the carpometacarpal joint of the thumb. In osteoarthritis of the other joints, genetic influences are less obvious. Secondary arthritis may follow sporting activities and trauma that produce recurrent traumatic synovitis.

Common problems treated with steroid injections

- *Osteoarthritis*: affecting the first carpometacarpal joint (thumb).
- *Rheumatoid arthritis*: acute exacerbations of the interphalangeal or carpometacarpal joints.
- *Carpal tunnel syndrome*: this is due to median nerve compression (nerve entrapment) at the wrist. This condition may be predisposed by conditions that cause weight increase, such as obesity, myxoedema, acromegaly, pregnancy, rheumatoid arthritis, collagen disorders, osteoarthritis and previous trauma affecting the bones of the wrist joint. The condition occurs more frequently in females and in those taking the oral contraceptive pill.
- *Tenosynovitis of the thumb (de Quervain's disease)*: the extensor pollicis brevis and the abductor pollicis longus tendons are particularly prone to inflammation following occupational trauma or repetitive stress.
- *Trigger finger*: this condition may be idiopathic but occurs more commonly in rheumatoid arthritis (it may be an early or late manifestation). It may affect any of the flexor tendon synovial sheaths in the palm, including the thumb.

The first carpometacarpal joint

The first carpometacarpal joint is one of the few joints affected by osteoarthritis in which the response to steroid injection is rewarding (the other joint responding well to steroid injection is the acromioclavicular joint). Commonly described as 'washerwomen's thumb', this type of osteoarthritis follows the repetitive chores undertaken in the course of domestic work.

Presentation and diagnosis

The patient commonly complains of aching around the joint, and examination reveals pain on passive backward movement of the thumb in extension. Often osteophytes are present, noted on X-ray examination of the joint. These may render injection into the small joint space difficult.

Functional anatomy

This joint is the articulation of the first metacarpal with the trapezium bone of the wrist. Extension and abduction of the thumb causes pain and there is deep tenderness in the 'anatomical snuffbox' at the joint line, which is more easily palpable when the subject flexes and tucks the thumb into the palm. The joint space, although small, will accept an injection of about 0.5 ml of steroid solution.

Injection technique (see Figure 4.1)

The patient tucks the thumb as far into the palm as possible and holds it there with the index and middle fingers. Palpate the joint line dorsally and then inject from the lateral aspect, taking care to avoid the abductor pollicis tendon as it marks the border of the snuffbox. Use a small $\frac{5}{8}$ inch (1.6 cm) needle and inject up to 0.5 ml triamcinolone acetonide. No lidocaine is required, although some doctors prefer to use an equal quantity of lidocaine 1% plain.

Metacarpal and interphalangeal joints

Acute exacerbations of rheumatoid arthritis affecting the small joints of the hands often benefit from direct injection of steroids such as triamcinolone acetonide, into the joint space or into the surrounding inflamed synovium and capsule.

Functional anatomy

These are simple joints, but it must be remembered that the joint space of the metacarpal joint is distal to the knuckle on palpation and is a condylar joint, with

Trapezium   Base of first metacarpal

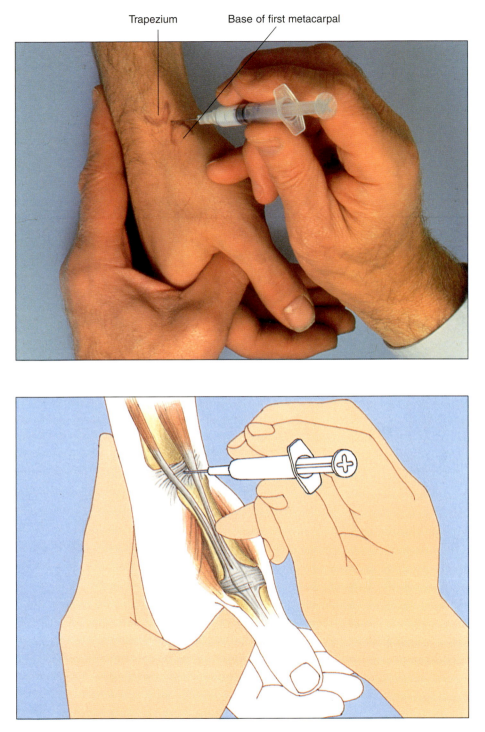

Figure 4.1 The first carpometacarpal joint.

one palmar and two collateral ligaments. The interphalangeal joints are simple hinge joints, each with a palmar and two collateral ligaments. It is important to remember the neurovascular bundle at the side of each joint when injecting.

Injection technique

Palpate the joint line often by applying some gentle traction to open up the joint space before injecting 0.25–0.5 ml triamcinolone acetonide anterolaterally into the joint space. As the joint spaces are so small, it is not necessary to mix the steroid with lidocaine unless the joints are very tender on palpation. Injection of two or three of these joints at a time is appropriate, and often a long-lasting remission of up to six months is attained.[1]

Carpal tunnel syndrome

Presentation and diagnosis

This is probably the most common nerve entrapment disorder, affecting women more commonly than men. It is caused by compression of the median nerve as it enters the palm posterior to the flexor retinaculum. The typical syndrome presents as pain radiating up the arm from the wrist, and paraesthesia affecting the median nerve distribution in the palm, namely the thumb, index and predominantly the middle finger and lateral half of the ring finger, paroxysmally affecting the patient in the night and being relieved on getting up and moving the arm and hand around. If left untreated, the condition may deteriorate and produce muscle wasting in the thenar eminence of the palm.

The middle finger is often the first and the worst finger to be affected by the paraesthesia. Occasionally the patient complains of paraesthesia affecting all the fingers of the hand, and this produces a diagnostic problem for the clinician. This may be due to a total entrapment of both the ulnar and median nerves. It is known that there may be anatomical connections between the ulnar and median nerves to account for this, and if the history is typical as described, a diagnosis of carpal tunnel syndrome may still confidently be made even though the patient complains of paraesthesia in all the fingers.

As described earlier, it is important to recognise and treat any of the predisposing or concomitant disorders in order to ensure a lasting recovery.

Tinel's test

This is a reliable diagnostic test. Percuss lightly over the flexor retinaculum with a tendon hammer, particularly between the palmaris longus tendon and the flexor carpi radialis tendons. The test is positive if the patient describes a tingling sensation in the median nerve distribution.

Phelan's test

This is another useful confirmatory test. Hold the wrist in acute flexion for up to one minute; this usually reproduces the pain and typical paraesthesia.

Diagnosis may be confirmed by electromyography, and this further test is recommended in cases of doubt. It is often necessary to exclude causes of paraesthesia in the hand or pain in the arm arising from the cervical spine, such as cervical disc lesions or spondylosis causing C5 or C6 nerve entrapments.

Functional anatomy

The median nerve lies posterior to the palmaris longus tendon at the wrist, and it enters the palm deep to the flexor retinaculum. The latter is a dense fibrous band covering the proximal one-third of the palm, into which the palmaris longus tendon is inserted. The palmaris longus tendon is the most central and superficial tendon, which is prominent when the wrist is flexed against resistance. Consequently, it is important to identify the palmaris longus tendon as this enables the operator to know the exact position of the median nerve. Approximately 13% of people do not possess a palmaris longus, in which case the median nerve is then identified as lying between the tendons of the flexor digitorum superficialis and the flexor carpi radialis. On entering the palm, the median nerve then lies in the carpal tunnel, where it divides into its digital branches.

Injection technique (see Figure 4.2)

Treatment of a mild carpal tunnel syndrome may initially be simple weight reduction advice together with a daily diuretic tablet, such as hydrochlorothiazide or cyclopenthiazide. Night splints may also help and may be the preferred management in early pregnancy. It is unwise to inject steroids in the first 16–18 weeks of pregnancy. If these simple measures are not successful, steroid injection is advisable and will be helpful in over 60% of cases. If there is no response to steroid injection (after two or three successive injections), or, very importantly if there is evidence of median nerve damage, such as thenar eminence muscle wasting, it is wise to refer for surgical decompression.

The patient sits facing the operator, with the palm of the affected hand facing upwards and resting on a firm surface. By flexing the wrist against resistance, the palmaris longus tendon is clearly seen. Make a thumbnail indentation or skin mark on the radial side of the tendon precisely at the distal crease of the wrist; this is the best injection site. As in all these procedures, it is kinder to the patient to inject, where possible, through a skin crease as this ensures less pain. If you cannot demonstrate the palmaris tendon, which is absent in 13% of patients, palpate the gap between the tendons of the flexor digitorum superficialis and the flexor carpi radialis and then mark the skin at the distal crease. Ensure that you avoid any surface veins.

Use 1 ml steroid, for example triamcinolone acetonide alone, in a 2 ml volume syringe. Use a 1 inch (2.5 cm) needle. No local anaesthetic is added, because its effect may cause an uncomfortable numbness in the fingers and palm in the median nerve distribution, lasting for several hours. The symptoms of carpal tunnel syndrome are very unpleasant for many patients, so reproducing these symptoms for several hours will produce much discomfort, not to mention causing some unpopularity for the doctor!

With the wrist now straight, advance the needle almost to the hilt, pointing distally and at an angle of 45 degrees. This ensures that the steroid solution is deposited in the carpal tunnel immediately behind the flexor retinaculum. At this moment, always ask the patient if this is comfortable and ensure that no pain is felt. Inadvertent needling of a digital branch of the median nerve will cause pain in the palm and referred along a finger. If this should occur, just withdraw the needle slightly before injecting. Aspirate to exclude any intravascular injection. You should then be able to inject the steroid easily, with little resistance to the plunger. Inject slowly, as this will ensure the least pain or discomfort produced by the injection.

The median nerve lies posterior to the palmaris longus tendon. If the needle insertion causes immediate paraesthesia, indicating that the needle has entered the substance of the median nerve, withdraw the needle slightly and reinsert it laterally. This will ensure that no damage is caused to the nerve itself.

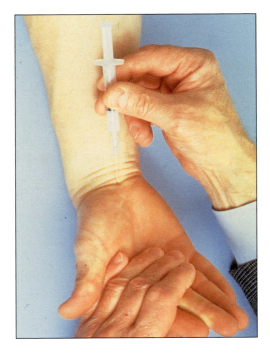

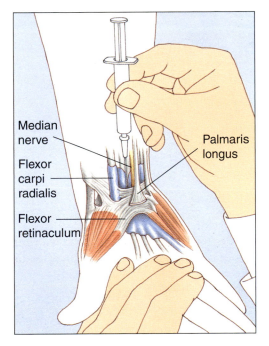

Median
nerve

Flexor
carpi
radialis

Flexor
retinaculum

Palmaris
longus

Figure 4.2 Carpal tunnel syndrome.

Always remember to remind the patient that some acute pain may be experienced for up to 48 hours after the injection. Advise that simple analgesia is effective, and instruct the patient to rest the arm for 24–48 hours after the injection.

Symptoms should resolve in the course of a few days, and reassurance is important. If the condition is bilateral, it is better to inject one side initially and await the clinical result. Sometimes the other side improves spontaneously and no further treatment is required. Where no improvement in symptoms is noted, a second injection about three weeks later is justified. However, where there is no improvement after three injections, it is wise to refer for surgical decompression.[2]

de Quervain's tenosynovitis

Presentation and diagnosis

This condition is usually due to repetitive strain, sports injury or occupational hazard. The patient complains of pain in the line of the tendon. On examination there may be some swelling and crepitus palpated on movement of the thumb. Diagnosis is confirmed by asking the patient to make a fist while flexing the thumb into the palm and ulnar-deviating the flexed wrist. This reproduces the pain. The pain also occurs on abduction and resisted extension of the thumb.

Functional anatomy

De Quervain's tenosynovitis affects the abductor pollicis longus and extensor pollicis brevis tendons, which have become inflamed. These tendons fuse as they cross the radial styloid and form a common synovial sheath which forms the anterior border of the 'snuffbox'. The tendons are lined with a synovial sheath, and in tenosynovitis the synovial surfaces become roughened, which causes pain and crepitus on movement of the tendon. In injecting, the aim is to introduce the steroid mixed with local anaesthetic into the space between the tendon and the sheath.

Injection technique (see Figure 4.3)

Use 1 ml steroid mixed with 1 ml lidocaine 1% plain in a 2 ml syringe, using a $\frac{5}{8}$ inch (1.6 cm) (number 20, 25 gauge) needle. Insert the needle along the line of the tendon just distal to the point of maximal tenderness, advancing it proximally into the substance of the tendon (it is more painful for the patient if this injection is introduced distally), when resistance to injection will be felt. Slowly withdraw the needle, while maintaining pressure on the plunger until the resistance disappears. At this point, the needle tip is in the tendon sheath and the whole 2 ml of solution may be injected. The sheath may visibly expand along its course as the solution is injected.

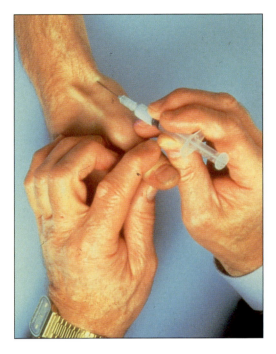

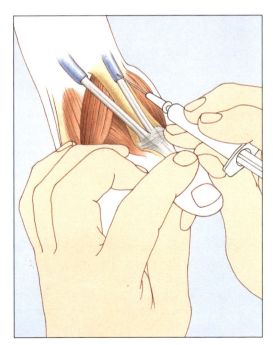

Figure 4.3 de Quervain's tenosynovitis.

One may select any of the steroids for this purpose. Relief of pain is usually dramatic and immediate.

Post-injection advice

It is wise to recommend a period of rest of the affected part for a few days and avoidance of painful movements or the tasks that initially caused the problem. Recurrences indicate that repetitive strain, possibly as a result of faulty technique, is the cause, and appropriate advice regarding occupation should be sought.

Trigger finger

Presentation and diagnosis

Trigger finger may be idiopathic but is common in early and late rheumatoid arthritis and affects any or all of the flexor tendons of the fingers in the palm. A tender nodule in the palm is usually palpated over the line of the flexor tendon just proximal to the metacarpophalangeal joint crease. Injection will be into the tendon sheath and not into this nodule. The patient complains of an uncomfortable locking of the affected finger spontaneously occurring in flexion; only with difficulty can the finger be released by manipulating or forcefully extending the affected joint. Naturally this condition is an occupational hazard for anyone undertaking machine or intricate work involving the hands and fingers.

Functional anatomy

This condition is a tenosynovitis affecting any of the flexor tendons (superficial and deep) in the palm. These tendons are enveloped by synovial sheaths as they traverse the carpal tunnel. They extend for about 1 inch (2.5 cm) above the flexor retinaculum to about halfway along each metacarpal, except for the little finger in which the sheath is continuous and extends to the terminal phalanx and the thumb (flexor pollicis longus), where the sheath is continuous to the tip of the finger. The fibrous synovial sheaths of the terminal parts of the tendons are thinner over the joints.

Injection technique (see Figure 4.4)

Use 1 ml steroid mixed with 1 ml lidocaine 1% plain in a 2 ml syringe with a $\frac{5}{8}$ inch (1.6 cm) needle. Insert the needle over the crease overlying the metacarpophalangeal joint and advance it proximally into the flexor tendon. Ask the

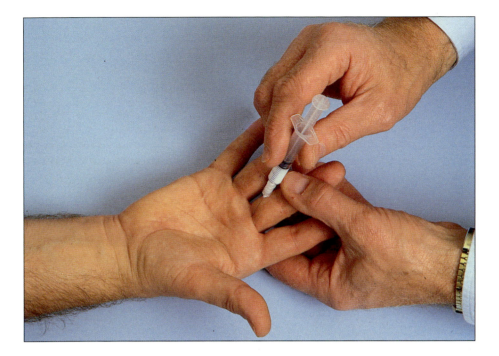

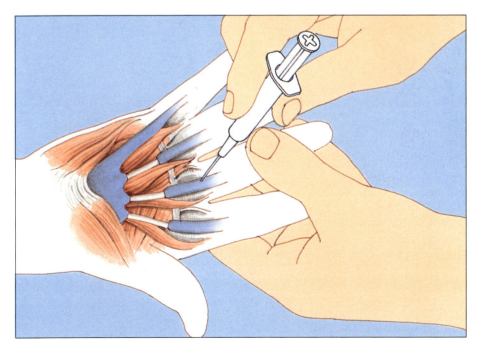

Figure 4.4 Trigger finger.

patient to flex that finger, which will move the needle, confirming that the needle point is in the tendon. Resistance to the plunger will be experienced. Slowly withdraw the needle while maintaining pressure on the plunger until resistance to injection disappears, when the contents may easily be injected into the tendon sheath. A slow injection of the solution will expand the part of the tendon sheath proximal to the injection, a confirmatory sign that the steroid is in the correct place.

It is important to emphasise that one should never attempt to inject steroid into the substance of a tendon. As stated previously, these injections should be easy with no force required, and the solution should just glide in.

Trigger fingers respond well to steroid injection but do recur and may be injected two to three times in a year if clinically required. However, further recurrences may need a surgical release.[3]

References

1   Raman J (2005) Intra-articular corticosteroid injection for first carpometacarpal osteoarthritis. *J Rheumatol.* **32**: 1305–6.

2   Agarwal V *et al* (2005) A prospective study of the long term efficacy of local methyl prednisolone acetate injection in the management of mild carpal tunnel syndrome. *Rheumatol.* **44**(5): 647–50.

3   Nimigan A *et al* (2006) Steroid injections in the management of trigger fingers. *Am J Phys Med Rehabil.* **85**(1): 36–43.

5 THE ELBOW

5 THE ELBOW

Perhaps the most common soft tissue lesions are those affecting the extensor and flexor insertions at the elbow, namely tennis and golfer's elbow, so called because the bad tennis forearm drive or the bad golf swing reputedly causes these conditions. In these lesions the tendon substance (tenoperiosteal junction), which has no synovial sheath, itself becomes inflamed and is a tendinitis and not a tenosynovitis, in which the tendon synovial sheath becomes inflamed.

Tennis elbow

Acute tennis elbow is common in young to middle-aged patients owing to strain of the extensor tendons of the forearm. Also known as lateral epicondylitis, it is a strain occurring at the tenoperiosteal insertion into the extensor epicondyle of the humerus. It is often caused by repetitive movements at work, such as screwdriving or polishing. A defective backhand or forehand drive at tennis, squash or badminton is often a causative factor.

Very rarely, a bony secondary deposit may cause pain and tenderness on palpation, which is not reproduced by resisted extension of the wrist. If in doubt, X-ray the elbow joint before injecting steroids.

Presentation and diagnosis

On palpation, there is exquisite pain and localised tenderness over the lateral epicondyle of the humerus. This pain may be reproduced by asking the patient to extend the hand at the wrist (dorsiflexion) against resistance. All other movements at the elbow are normal.

Functional anatomy

The common insertion of the extensor muscles of the forearm and the hand is the lateral epicondyle of the humerus. These muscles are essentially the brachioradialis, extensor carpi radialis, extensor carpi ulnaris and digitorum muscles. Strain of any of these muscles at their insertion will cause a tendinitis at this site, which will produce an easily localised point of acute tenderness. Asking the patient to extend the wrist against resistance enables the operator to pinpoint the lesion accurately.

Injection technique

Use 1 ml steroid in a 2 ml syringe with a $\frac{5}{8}$ inch (1.6 cm) needle. Personal choice will dictate whether or not to mix the steroid with local anaesthetic. It is important to remember that local anaesthetic, such as lidocaine, will prevent the discovery of all the tender points of the lesion as it is so effective. Using steroid alone is more painful for the patient, but the overall success of the injection is higher because the operator will be able to detect all the painful or tender parts of the lesion.

Success depends on identifying and infiltrating all the points of tenderness in the tenoperiosteal junction at one injection. First locate the point of maximal tenderness with the patient, extending the hand against your resistance; then make a thumbnail indentation at the needle entry point. After inserting the needle in a proximal direction (*see* Figure 5.1), ask the patient each time whether the needle is in a tender spot, moving the needle around the lesion in a clockwise direction and in a fan shape subcutaneously after the initial skin puncture and ensuring that all tender points are injected accurately with about 0.1–0.2 ml steroid each time, delivering in all up to 1 ml steroid. This may be described as a 'pepper pot' technique (*see* Figure 5.2).

Using this technique of infiltrating all the tender parts of the tendinitis lesion, one can be more assured of complete success in treating tennis and golfer's elbow and also lessening the frequently reported recurrences.

The patient may sit or lie down during this procedure and must be warned that the pain of the injection may persist for up to 48 hours but should then subside. Simple analgesia may be advised. The arm should be rested for a day or two after the injection. Patients should be advised not to carry bags and shopping with the affected arm for a week or so after the injection.

Golfer's elbow

This condition mirrors the lesion of tennis elbow, occurring in the origin of the forearm flexor muscles at the medial epicondyle of the humerus. Also known as medial epicondylitis, it may be due to the golf player's faulty backswing and to other repetitive movements affecting the flexor muscle group.

Presentation and diagnosis

The patient complains of acute tenderness on a spot over the medial epicondyle, which is easily reproduced at this site by asking the patient to flex the hand at the wrist against resistance.

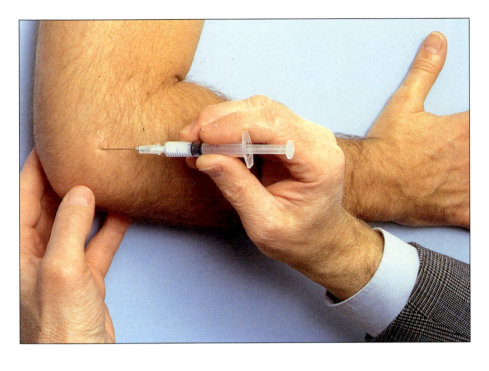

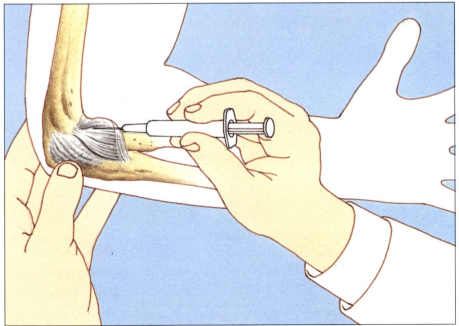

Figure 5.1 Tennis elbow.

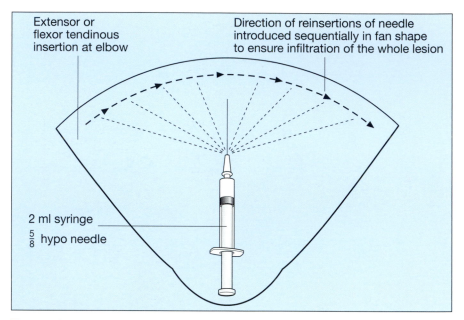

Figure 5.2 Lateral or medial epicondyle elbow.

Functional anatomy

The common tendon insertion of the muscles of the flexor group at the medial epicondyle is affected. They are the flexor carpi radialis, digitorum superficialis, flexor carpi ulnaris and palmaris longus. As in tennis elbow, the lesion is localised to the tenoperiosteal junction. It is important to recall that the ulnar nerve is in close proximity in the canal posterior to the medial epicondyle and may be punctured easily by the injecting needle. Prior to the injection, when the needle is *in situ*, the doctor should confirm that no paraesthesiae are felt in the ulnar distribution, i.e. in the little finger and the ulnar side of the ring finger.

Injection technique (see Figure 5.3)

The patient sits with his back to the operator or lies on a couch with the fore-arm of the affected side behind the back and the dorsum of the hand resting on the buttock. The tender spot in the medial epicondyle is identified by asking the patient to flex the hand against resistance. Mark the spot with a thumbnail indentation as the site of needle entry.

Use 1 ml steroid in a 2 ml syringe with a $\frac{5}{8}$ inch (1.6 cm) needle and proceed to infiltrate all the tender spots of the lesion precisely as described above for treating tennis elbow (*see* Figure 5.2).

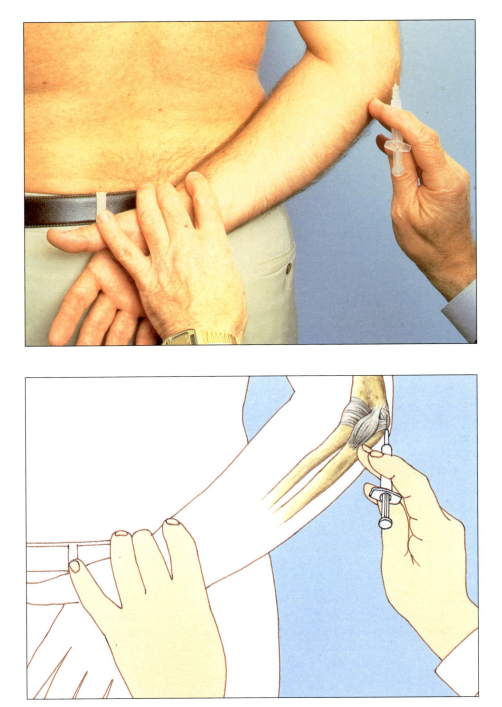

Figure 5.3 Golfer's elbow.

Post-injection advice

This is essential, as for tennis elbow. Avoid the painful movements for the next few days after the injection. Remember that there may be 'after pain' for up to 48 hours, after which the condition is expected to improve. Simple analgesic tablets may be all that is required for a day or so. Repeat injections may be given at three- or four-weekly intervals, up to a total of three injections in 12 months if necessary.

Lipodystrophy

Remember that both tennis and golfer's elbow are superficial lesions and the injection must be made deeply into the fibrous substance of the tenoperiosteal junction. This effectively means that the needle point may well touch the periosteum. If this is not ensured, it is all too easy to inject steroid into the subcutaneous fat, in which case dimpling of the skin due to fat dissolution may occur. It is always wise when injecting these lesions to warn the patient beforehand of this possibility in order to minimise any future complaint of negligence. The more potent intra-articular steroids have the reputation of causing lipodystrophy; but any steroid preparation injected into the subcutaneous fat layer may produce it.

Olecranon bursitis (see Figure 5.4)

This condition is one of several painful bursae problems commonly occurring in general practice. It may occur following repeated minor trauma and is also known as 'student's elbow'. It may also occur in gout and should be investigated when there is no other obvious cause. In rheumatoid disease, nodules may be palpable in this bursa. In gout, tophi may be present.

The synovial tissue behind the elbow joint and the olecranon process is quite profuse and lax, and commonly a bursa filled with clear, yellow, viscous effusion appears. The swelling appears and often enlarges in size, and can be quite tense and fluctuant on palpation. Sometimes the bursa is reddened with acute sepsis, which may require antibiotic therapy. There is, however, more often no obvious infection and aspiration is a simple matter. A 1.5 inch (3.8 cm) needle is inserted into the bursa and the fluid aspirated using a 10 ml syringe. Occasionally these bursae may be loculated, and it is necessary to move the needle point around within the bursa to completely evacuate the serous contents.

Microscopy may reveal polymorphonuclear leucocytes in infection or urate crystals in gout. A firm Tubigrip bandage should be applied afterwards to prevent the bursa refilling. Repeated aspiration may be necessary. In frequent recurrences, it is helpful to inject these with 1 ml steroid after aspiration, with a fair chance of preventing the recurrence of the condition.

Following injection and aspiration, apply a firm elastic or double Tubigrip support around the elbow. This may help prevent the bursa refilling with fluid.

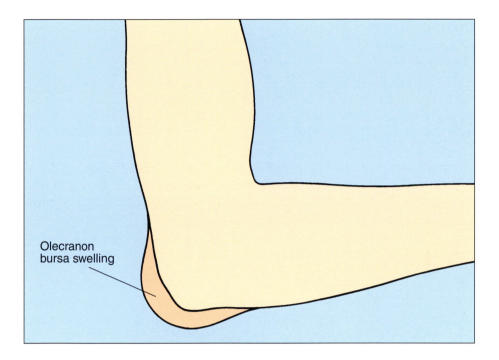

Olecranon bursa swelling

Figure 5.4 Olecranon bursitis.

Elbow joint

Presentation

Painful elbow occurs in exacerbations of arthritis and post-traumatic synovitis (e.g following the unaccustomed carrying of heavy objects such as luggage with the arm extended). All movements of flexion, pronation and supination aggravate the pain.

Functional anatomy

The elbow joint comprises the trochlea of the humerus, articulating with the trochlear notch of the ulna (olecranon) in addition to the articulation of the radial head with lower end of the humerus (the capitulum). The synovial membrane is extensive and forms a soft palpable pad together with extrasynovial fat, anteriorly. Injection of the joint is easiest by palpating anterolaterally into this soft pad, using the finger to determine the bone edges between the lateral epicondyle of the humerus, the olecranon process and the head of radius. A triangle is formed, the centre of which is the best point for needle insertion. Gentle passive movement of the forearm and the radial head by pronating and supinating reveals the joint space outline and facilitates the injection.

Injection technique

Sit the patient, with the forearm at an angle of 90 degrees, resting on the examination couch or a table. Make a thumbnail imprint at the point of injection, as above, resting the examining finger on an alcohol swab. Insert the needle in an anterolateral direction for 1–2 cm and slowly inject a solution of steroid such as triamcinalone acetonide 1 ml mixed with 1–3 ml lidocaine plain 1%, using a blue hub 1 inch (2.5 cm) needle. The injection should be quite easy and free. If resistance to injection is noticed then gently move the needle slightly until completion is easy.

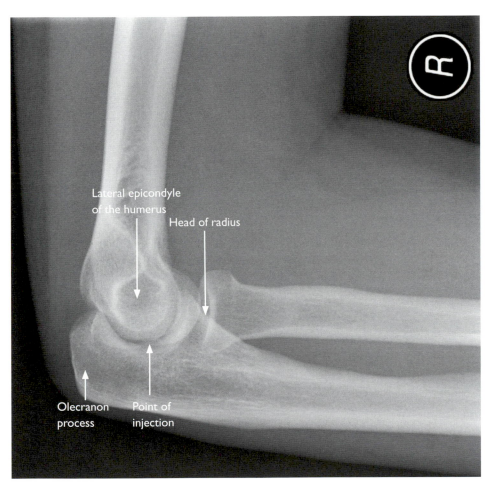

Figure 5.5 Right elbow, lateral view

6 CONDITIONS AROUND THE HIP AND THIGH

6 CONDITIONS AROUND THE HIP AND THIGH

The hip

Steroid injections into the hip joint are not nowadays commonly performed. The procedure is more complicated than for other intra-articular injections, and it is not advisable for general practitioners to undertake it. Moreover, the management of osteoarthritis of the hip joint has radically changed in the last few years because of the success of hip replacement operations and the marked improvement of the hip prostheses that are now fitted. However, there are several conditions that are easily treated in the practice.

Trochanteric bursitis

This may occur in rheumatoid arthritis or following minor trauma. The patient complains of pain around the hip. On further enquiry, it is apparent that the pain is felt laterally over the greater trochanter of the femur, worse when lying on the affected side in bed at night. The bursa is fluctuant on palpation and is often multilocular and situated over the posterolateral surface of the greater trochanter and gluteus maximus muscle.

Consensus opinions of orthopaedic physicians and sports medicine specialists have recently suggested that trochanteric bursitis should be better known as greater trochanter pain syndrome (GTPS).[1]

It is postulated that the significant short-term superiority of a single cortico-steroid injection over home training and shockwave therapy declines after one month. This condition is a painful overuse syndrome of the hip in adults engaging in recreational sports activities. The anatomical relationship between three bursae, the hip adductor–external rotator muscles, the greater trochanter and the overlying iliotibial tract (band), may predispose this area to biomechanical irritation. Magnetic resonance imaging (MRI) studies have shown abnormalities that appear to better correlate with the GTPS than any other bursal lesion. These studies showed swellings of the trochanteric bursa to be uncommon – hence the suggestion to label all these conditions of pain around the lateral hip joint as greater trochanteric pain syndrome.

Injection technique (see Figure 6.1)

The patient lies on the couch with the affected side uppermost and the hip flexed. At the most tender spot over the trochanter, perpendicularly insert a 1 inch (2.5 cm) needle attached to a 10 ml syringe, until the bone is reached. Withdraw the needle slightly and aspirate the clear yellow fluid. Then, leaving the needle *in situ*, change the syringe so that 1 ml steroid may be injected into the bursa and the tough fibrous insertion of the gluteal fascia.

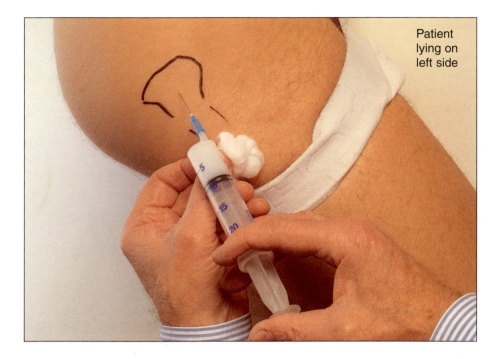

Patient lying on left side

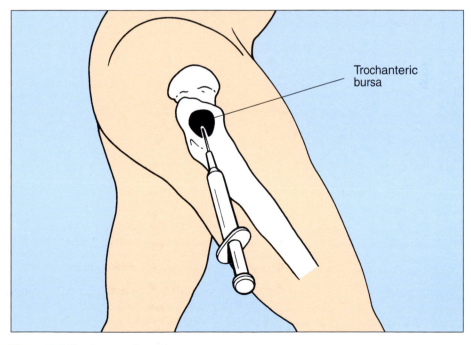

Trochanteric bursa

Figure 6.1 Trochanteric bursitis.

Ischiogluteal bursitis

This condition is characterised by pain felt deeply in the buttock over the ischial tuberosity and aggravated by sitting, especially on hard surfaces. The medial area of this bony prominence is covered with fibro-fatty substance that contains the ischial bursa of the gluteus maximus muscle. The bursa lies over the ischial tuberosity and the sciatic nerve. Because of the deep-seated pain experienced, it is often confused with sciatic pain, making a difficult differential diagnosis. On examination, straight leg raising is usually normal, but there is tenderness felt deeply in the buttock on palpation, and it may be possible to detect a fluctuant swelling.

Prolonged sitting on hard surfaces or a bicycle saddle may precipitate the condition.

Injection technique (see Figure 6.2)

With the patient lying prone or on the side with the hip flexed and the affected side uppermost, inject 1 ml steroid mixed with 1 ml lidocaine 1% plain in a 2 ml syringe into the point of maximal tenderness. It is necessary to use a larger, 1.5 inch (3.8 cm), needle to reach the bursa. When the injection has been sited correctly, the pain and tenderness will be abolished immediately, on account of the local anaesthetic; this confirms that the diagnosis was indeed the correct one.

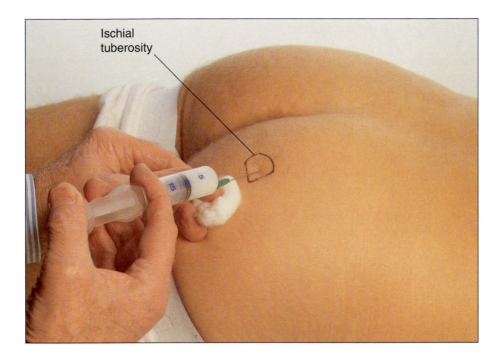

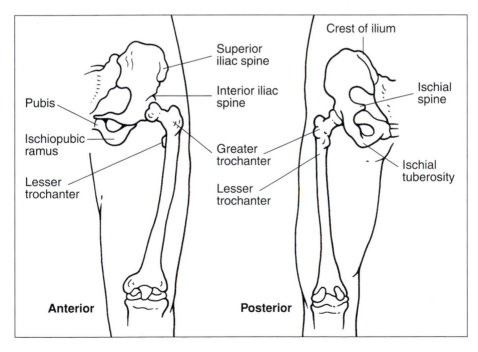

Figure 6.2 Ischiogluteal bursitis.

Meralgia paraesthetica

This entrapment syndrome is due to compression of the lateral cutaneous nerve of the thigh as it passes through the deep fascia about 3.9 inches (10 cm) below and medial to the anterior superior crest of the iliac spine. The nerve supplies the anterior and lateral surfaces of the mid-thigh. Typical paraesthesiae are felt in the front and side of the thigh, often after walking or prolonged standing. Usually occurring in overweight patients, the condition may be affected by a change in posture. Examination often reveals an area of numbness on the front of the thigh and bluntness to pinprick, and the diagnosis is confirmed by palpating the point of local tenderness where the nerve enters the thigh.

Early presentation of this syndrome may be mistaken for the initial stages of a Herpes zoster infection and it may be wise to wait for two weeks before injecting.

Injection technique (see Figure 6.3)

Locate the tender spot in the upper thigh 3.9 inches (10 cm) below and medial to the anterior superior iliac spine. Using a 2 ml syringe with a 1 inch (2.5 cm) needle and 1 ml steroid mixed with 1 ml lidocaine 1% plain, carefully infiltrate the solution around this spot.

Advice regarding posture and weight reduction is useful in preventing recurrences of the condition. Chronic cases occasionally require surgical referral for division of the lateral cutaneous nerve.

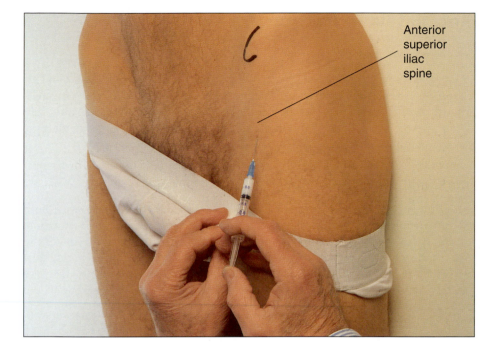

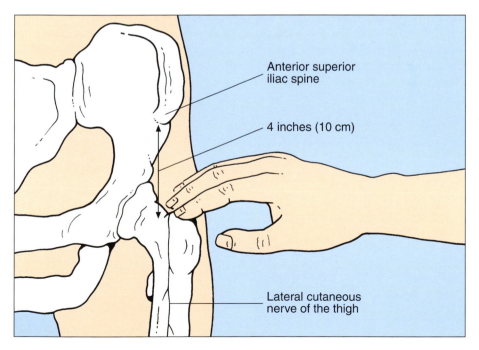

Figure 6.3 Meralgia paraesthetica.

Iliotibial band friction syndrome

Presentation and diagnosis

This overuse injury is commonly seen in long distance runners, cyclists and ski-ers and occasionally in golfers and walkers. Males are more commonly affected. Pain occurs at the lateral side of the knee joint superior to the joint line and often radiates up the lateral side of the thigh. There is a point of maximal tenderness over the lateral femoral condyle.

Functional anatomy

The iliotibial band is a thickening of the fascia lata in the lateral side of the thigh. It is superficial and extends from the anterior superior iliac spine to the tubercle (Gurdy) on the anterolateral side of the upper tibia. Flexion and extension of the knee joint causes the band to move in an anterior and posterior fashion, thus causing friction of the band over the lateral femoral condyle. Pain may be quite acute, which is an indication to inject steroid. Otherwise physiotherapy in the form of deep massage, heat and anti-inflammatories are useful.

Injection technique (see Figure 6.4)

Inject 0.5–1 ml of hexacetonide or methylprednisolone acetate (Depo-Medrone®) mixed with 0.5–1 ml lidocaine 1% plain, using a 1 inch (2.5 cm) blue hub needle at the point of maximal tenderness, over the lateral side of the femoral condyle, after making a thumbnail imprint to identify the point of injection. Occasionally a bursa is present posterior to the insertion, and it should be injected.

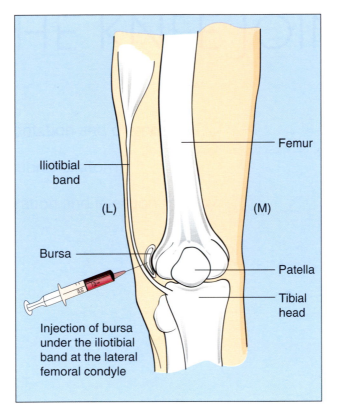

Figure 6.4 Iliotibial band syndrome.

Reference

1   Rompe JD *et al* (2009) Home training, local corticosteroid injection, or radial shock wave therapy for greater trochanter pain syndrome. *Am J Sports Med*. 37(10): 1981–90.

7 THE KNEE JOINT

Effusions of the knee joint are commonly seen in general practice, and both aspiration and steroid injection may be confidently undertaken.

There are many causes of effusion, such as trauma, strained collateral ligaments, cruciate and meniscus tears, haemarthrosis, rheumatoid disease, osteoarthritis, Reiter's syndrome, gout, pseudogout, psoriasis and, rarely, chondromalacia patellae.

Prepatellar and infrapatellar bursae ('clergyman's' and 'housemaid's' knees), occur because of recurrent pressure or trauma of kneeling and should not be confused with effusion of the knee joint. Prepatellar bursitis was more common in coal miners and in carpet layers. These latter are prone to infection and must be distinguished from effusion of the knee joint. Osteochondritis dissecans causing loose bodies in the knee joint may lead to effusion and locking of the joint. Baker's cyst posteriorly may rupture during violent flexion of the joint. This may occur in rheumatoid arthritis.

Presentation and diagnosis

An effusion is often detected on inspection and both knees should be inspected with the patient first standing and then lying on the couch.

Palpate the patella for the following signs:

- with an effusion, the hollows alongside the kneecap disappear, and a suprapatellar bulge may appear that is painful on palpation. The 'patella tap' may be less painful with smaller effusions, but the fluid can be stroked from one side of the patella to the other
- synovial thickening, which may be nodular, indicates synovitis
- bony prominences (osteophytes), which may occur in osteoarthritis
- note the temperature, by placing the backs of the fingers on the patella. In infection and crystal synovitis, there will be warmth, tenderness and redness of the overlying skin
- patellar 'grating' and crepitus, which occur in osteoarthritis.

Examine the full active and passive movements of the knee joint and note any quadriceps wasting.

It is known that hyaluronan (hyaluronic acid) in synovial fluid is responsible for absorbing mechanical shocks, producing elastoviscous protection for soft tissues, shielding pain receptors and protecting cartilage against inflammatory mediators and degradative enzymes. Viscosupplementation is a means of injecting into the knee joint hyaluronic acid preparations of high molecular weight with optimal elastoviscous properties. These have the effect of restoring osteoarthritis synovial fluid to healthy levels and reducing pain and improving mobility. There are several preparations on the market – hylan G-F 20 (Synvisc®) in the UK and hyaluronic acid (Hyalgan®) in Europe. The former product has a higher molecular weight than the latter and claims a superior clinical effect.

Treatment using hylan G-F 20 is by administering a course of three intra-articular injections over three weeks. This course may be repeated, the maximum dose being six injections in six months. Adverse events are rare and transient and the average duration of effective relief is 8.2 months following one course of three injections. It is therefore worth considering for use in patients not helped by, or suffering adverse effects of, NSAID therapy.[2] Patients awaiting knee replacement surgery may also well be supported by this therapy and for some patients it may even delay the need for surgery.

Adverse effects of viscosupplementation

After injection, increased pain and swelling may occur in approximately 2% of patients and may last up to a few days.

Always send joint aspirate for microscopy and analysis, for diagnosis and to exclude infection. Joint aspirate in normal patients should appear clear and pale yellow in colour. Any turbidity in appearance of the joint aspirate will be suspicious of infection, in which case steroids must not be injected until the pathology laboratory excludes infection.

Analysis of the synovial fluid will usually confirm the diagnosis. A summary of the diagnostic signs is shown in Table 7.1.

Inject with steroids no more than once every three months. This is most effective for acute flare-ups of arthropathy, especially those that affect a single joint, as in psoriasis or rheumatoid arthritis exacerbations. Unlike steroids, a viscosupplementation course of three injections in three weeks may be repeated twice in one year.

Technique of aspiration and injection (see Figure 7.1)

The patient lies on the couch with the knee slightly flexed; a pillow behind the knee is helpful. This allows relaxation of the quadriceps and patellar tendon. Carefully palpate the bony margin of the patella, which may be moved freely before the needle is inserted. Injection can be from either the lateral or the medial side of the patella and below the superior border of the patella.

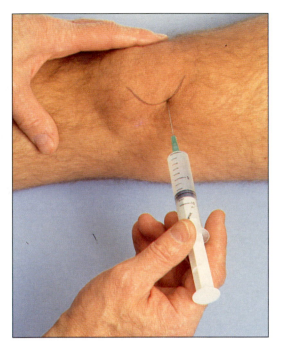

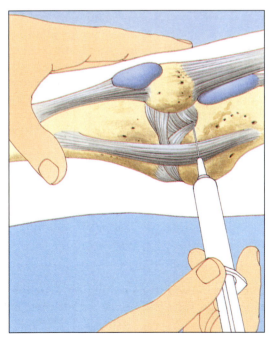

Figure 7.1 The knee joint.

Aspiration

- Prepare a 20 ml (or 50 ml) volume syringe and a sterile specimen container for diagnostic microscopy and culture. Use a 1.5 inch (3.8 cm) needle.
- Insert the needle horizontally and in a slightly downward (or posterior) direction into the joint, in the gap between the back of the patella and the femoral condyles. When the needle is behind the patella, it is in the joint space. Just before reaching that stage, it should be possible to slide the patella over the femur freely from side to side, ensuring relaxation of the quadriceps.
- If a steroid injection is to follow the aspiration, leave a small amount of synovial fluid in the knee joint. This will allow the steroid to diffuse around the joint cavity more easily.
- It is kinder, but not strictly necessary, to infiltrate 1 ml lidocaine 1% plain into the skin at the aspiration site.

Injection

- Use 1 ml steroid (20 mg triamcinolone acetonide, 40 mg methylprednisolone or 20 mg hydrocortisone acetate) in a 2 ml volume syringe. Use a 1.5 inch (3.8 cm) needle.
- Follow the same needle insertion procedure as for aspiration, above.
- Inject steroid into the knee no more than once every three months. After aspiration or injection, the knee joint should be rested for 24 hours, supported by a firm Tubigrip or elastic crêpe bandage.

The short-term benefit of intra-articular steroids in the treatment of osteoarthritis of the knee joint is well established and few side-effects have been reported. Longer-term beneficial effects have not been confirmed.

The response to hyaluronan appears to be more durable.[3–6]

References

1 Balaz EA and Denliger JL (1993) Viscosupplementation: a new concept in the treatment of os teoarthritis. *J Rheumatol.* **20**(39): 3–9.

2 Dickson DJ and Hosie G (1998) Poster at BSR conference, Brighton.

3 Bellamy N *et al* (2006) Intra-articular corticosteroid for treatment of osteoarthritis of the knee. *Cochrane Database Syst Rev.* **2**: CD005328.

4 Bagga H *et al* (2006) Long-term effects of intra-articular hyaluronan on synovial fluid in osteoarthritis of the knee. *J Rheumatol.* **33**: 946–50.

5 Petrella RJ and Petrella M (2006) A prospective, randomized, double-blind, placebo controlled study to evaluate the efficacy of intra-articular hyaluronic acid for osteoarthritis of the knee. *J Rheumatol.* **33**: 951–6.

6 Gossec L and Dougados M (2006) Do intra-articular therapies work and who will benefit most? *Best Pract Res Clin Rheumatol.* **20**: 131–44.

8 THE ANKLE AND FOOT

8 THE ANKLE AND FOOT

Disorders of the foot and ankle are increasingly common in general practice owing to the popularity of sports and physical training, in particular jogging. Ankle sprains, the most common injury in general practice, have an estimated episode rate of 28 per 2500 patients per year.

Functional anatomy

The ankle joint is a simple hinge joint, allowing only simple plantar and dorsiflexion. The joint is supported by a fibrous capsule, a lateral (calcaneofibular) and a medial (deltoid) ligament, and anterior and posterior ligaments. The tibialis anterior muscle, assisted by the extensor digitorum longus and extensor hallucis longus, account for dorsiflexion. Plantar flexion is brought about by the gastrocnemius and soleus, assisted by the plantaris, tibialis posterior, flexor hallucis longus and flexor digitorum longus muscles. The other main movements of the foot are eversion and inversion, which take place at the talocalcaneal, talonavicular and calcaneocuboid joints. The latter two together form the mid-tarsal joint. The forefoot, involving the heads of the metatarsals, is the site of many painful conditions, known collectively as metatarsalgia.

Presentation of some common problems

- *Lateral ligament sprains*: sprains as a result of inversion injury cause a complete or partial tear of the lateral ligament. Pain and swelling may be considerable, leading to difficulty in accurate assessment of the damage.
- *Achilles tendon*: rupture is characterised by sudden and severe pain in the calf (as if being suddenly kicked from behind), in the absence of any obvious injury. The tear may be palpated and the patient is unable to stand on the toes of the affected foot. Immediate referral for suture or immobilisation is indicated. Achilles tendinitis is caused by inflammation of the tendon at the insertion into the calcaneum or along the length of the tendon, or in the bursa separating the tendon from the calcaneum. Crepitus may be felt, as in any other form of tenosynovitis. The popularity of jogging has increased the incidence

of these problems. It should be noted that tendon inflammation and rupture are a recognised complication, occurring rarely, during therapy with some quinolone antibiotics, e.g. ciprofloxacin. The reason for this is not understood, but I can confirm from personal experience, the rupture of two posterior tibial tendons and one Achilles tendon following medication with ciprofloxacin. In any patient considered to be prone to tendinosis problems or similar tenosynovitis problems, avoidance of such antibiotic prescription must be advised.[1]

- *Plantar fasciitis*: this painful heel condition is characterised by an acutely tender spot in the middle of the heel pad on standing or walking. There is often a calcaneal spur demonstrated on an X-ray of the heel. This condition may occur in the seronegative arthropathies and should be suspected if the X-ray also demonstrates erosions or a fluffy or irregular calcaneal spur.
- *Tarsal tunnel syndrome*: this is an uncommon condition of posterior tibial nerve entrapment as it passes under the flexor retinaculum, and is analogous to the carpal tunnel syndrome of the wrist. The patient will complain of paroxysmal paraesthesia, numbness and pain along the medial border of the foot, the great toe and the distal part of the sole.
- *The ankle and mid-tarsal joint*: the ankle and the mid-tarsal joint may be affected by rheumatoid arthritis, the subtalar joint being more commonly affected. Seronegative arthropathies, such as Reiter's syndrome, psoriasis and ankylosing spondylitis, may affect the small mid-tarsal joints of the foot.
- *The forefoot*: this is involved in the many causes of metatarsalgia, especially pes cavus, March fracture, hallux rigidus and Morton's neurofibroma. Also in the elderly, the fatty pad of the sole may degenerate, causing the patient to complain that it is like 'walking on marbles'. Rheumatoid arthritis and gout may affect the forefoot, the latter condition most commonly affecting the first metatarsal joint of the great toe. Toe deformities such as hallux rigidus, hammer toes, claw toes and bunions all cause metatarsalgia.

Injection technique

Ankle sprains

These are best treated with the standard management of 'RICE': rest, ice, compression and elevation. This will help to provide pain relief and reduce inflammation and swelling. Physiotherapy referral is appropriate. Many doctors practising sports medicine will, if pain and swelling are severe, inject with local anaesthetic such as lidocaine 1% plain or bupivacaine (Marcain® plain) 0.25 or 0.5%, in addition to a steroid such as triamcinolone acetonide, methylprednisolone or hydrocortisone acetate, into the site of maximum tenderness (*see* Figure 8.1).

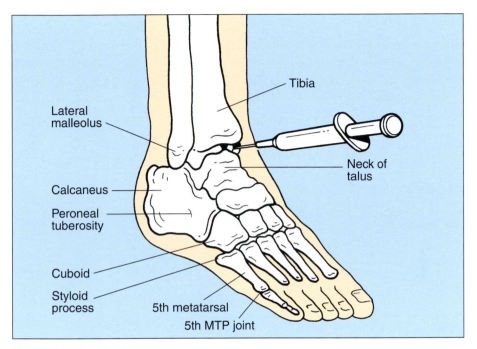

Figure 8.1 The ankle joint.

Achilles tendon

Although steroid injections are useful in Achilles bursitis and, with extreme caution, in Achilles tendinitis, general practitioners (GPs) are well advised to refrain from this treatment. The relief is so often only temporary and the possibility of Achilles tendon rupture so likely that the advice is to refer these problems for specialist care. Unfortunately the incidence of litigation is high, and GPs are best advised to diagnose Achilles tendon problems with care, never to inject steroid into the substance of a tendon and preferably to seek the advice of a specialist in these cases.

Plantar fasciitis: the painful heel

The painful heel is an acutely tender spot in the middle of the heel pad, which can be accurately palpated by firm pressure. The pain is due to plantar fasciitis, which is a strain of the long plantar ligament at its insertion into the calcaneum. The condition may occur alone or in other forms of arthritis such as Reiter's disease and ankylosing spondylitis.

Injection technique (see Figure 8.2)

Use 1 ml triamcinolone acetonide mixed with lidocaine (1% plain) in a 2 ml volume syringe with a 1 inch (2.5 cm) needle.

Allow the patient to lie prone on the examination couch with the heel facing uppermost. First swab the area to be injected liberally with 70% alcohol.

Although the skin of the heel is thicker and tougher on the plantar surface, it is better to inject from the centre of the heel pad rather than from the side of the heel pad (where the skin is thinner). This will ensure more accurate localisation of the injection. Infiltrate the skin and subcutaneous area with 1% lidocaine plain and infiltrate lidocaine deeply down to the calcaneal spur, and then change the syringe leaving the needle *in situ*; the tip of the needle is accurately placed at the point of maximum tenderness, often touching the periosteum, before 0.5– 1 ml of steroid mixed with 1 ml 1% lidocaine solution is injected. The whole lesion should preferably be infiltrated by moving the needle point to each tender spot to cover the whole lesion – as described for tennis elbow.

Since this is a painful injection, it is best to mix the steroid solution with lidocaine and infiltrate the skin as much as possible, while at the same time advancing the needle towards the most tender spot. As the duration of action of lidocaine is only between two and four hours, bupivacaine plain 0.25% or 0.5% may be used instead of the lidocaine in recurrent cases. As the duration of action of bupivacaine may last for up to 16 hours, it is often kinder for the patient in order to ensure an anaesthetic effect until the anti-inflammatory effect of the steroid takes over.

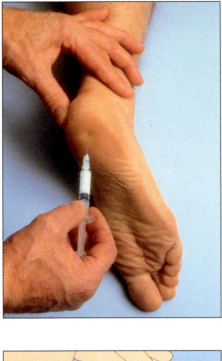

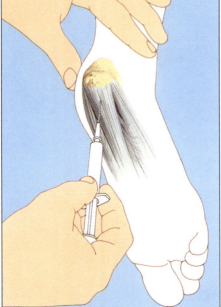

Figure 8.2 The painful heel.

Simple analgesia, avoiding walking on the affected heel for a couple of days and perhaps wearing a sponge rubber heel pad for a few days is sound post-injection advice.

Tarsal tunnel syndrome

This condition may also be treated with steroid injection, as for carpal tunnel syndrome in the wrist. The needle is inserted posterior to the flexor retinaculum behind the medial malleolus, between that and the calcaneus of the ankle joint.

The ankle joint

The anterior approach to injection and aspiration is the simplest and the only approach that GPs should adopt. Flare-ups of arthropathies respond well to injection of this joint. Care must be scrupulously exercised to avoid infection.

Injection technique

Insert the needle into the space between the tibia and the talus anteriorly, and between the tibialis anterior and the extensor hallucis longus tendons; 1 ml steroid mixed with 1 ml lidocaine 1% plain may be injected using a 1 inch (2.5 cm) needle. As for the knee joint, any aspirate should be sent for microscopy and analysis. Strict aseptic precautions must be adhered to as the ankle joint is particularly prone to infection.

In addition to corticosteroid injection for osteoarthritis of the ankle joint, visco-supplementation, using sodium hyaluronate, has been found to be effective. The latter will provide sustained relief of pain and improve ankle function.[2]

Posterior tibial tendinitis

This strain is due to a tenosynovitis of the tendon sheath. Usually a sports injury, e.g. in footballers, it may also be caused by a simple strain such as working on a ladder and reaching on a plantar flexed foot. It may also occur in rheumatoid arthritis. The pain is reproduced by inversion of the plantar flexed foot. Crepitus may be palpable along the line of the tendon sheath, especially directly posterior and inferior to the medial malleolus.

Functional anatomy

This muscle arises from the lateral part of the posterior surface of the tibia, the interosseous membrane and the adjoining part of the fibula. It is thus the deepest muscle in the calf. The tendon then becomes more superficial and grooves

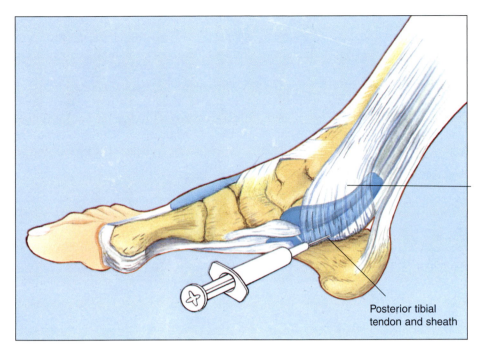

Posterior tibial
tendon and sheath

Figure 8.3 Posterior tibial tendinitis.

the posterior surface of the lower end of the tibia and lies behind and directly below the medial malleolus. It then passes forward under the flexor retinaculum into the sole of the foot. It is inserted into the tuberosity of the navicular bone and gives off slips which pass to the calcaneum, the cuboid, the three cuneiform bones and the bases of the second, third and fourth metatarsals.

A strain of this tendon may produce pain in the ankle and foot anywhere along the course of the tendon or any of its attachments in the foot.

Injection technique (see Figure 8.3)

Use a small needle $\frac{5}{8}$ inch (1.6 cm) with a 2 ml syringe containing 0.5–1.0 ml triamcinolone acetonide mixed with 1 ml lidocaine 1% plain. Place the fingers of the left hand on the tendon sheath immediately behind the medial malleolus to steady the tendon, and inject the needle in line with the tendon below the medial malleolus and in a proximal direction. As in the earlier descriptions of other forms of tenosynovitis injection, it is preferable to place the needle deeply into the substance of the tendon, when the doctor will immediately notice resistance to the injection. Then, while maintaining pressure on the syringe plunger, as if to inject, gradually withdraw the needle and syringe until the moment that no resistance to injection is felt – the needle is now in the tendon sheath space. Then inject up to 2 ml of the mixture.

It is helpful for the patient to rest the foot and ankle for a few days after the injection and to wear an elastic ankle support for up to six weeks. The only physiotherapy adjunct to treatment that is helpful is deep friction twice weekly for three or four weeks.

References

1 *ABPI Compendium of Data Sheets and Summaries of Product Characteristics 1999–2000 with the Code of Practice for the Pharmaceutical Industry*. Datapharm Publication, London, p. 167.

2 Salk R *et al* (2005) Viscosupplementation (hyaluronans) in the treatment of ankle osteoarthritis. *Clin Podiatr Med Surg N Am*. **22**: 585–97.

9 THE SPINE

9 THE SPINE

Painful conditions in the cervical, dorsal and lumbar spine are very common problems presenting to the general practitioner (GP). Careful history and examination is necessary to determine the true nature of the problem and to make an accurate diagnosis.

The commonest causes of back pain are those due to muscle and spinal ligament strains and will be treated by accepted clinical procedures. Conditions such as disc lesions and root pain will be similarly treated by standard practice.

Other causes of pain in the neck, scapula and lumbar areas are often less specific and may be due to facet (apophyseal) joint locking or to areas of acute localised tenderness in the superficial muscles. Facet joint problems can usually be easily diagnosed and are likely to cause pain on hyperextension of the lumbar spine. In the dorsal spine facet, joint lesions are characterised by acute tenderness felt at the affected level on full flexion of the neck. Facet joint lesions are best treated by manipulation, mobilisation techniques and other types of physiotherapy. It is known that the capsule of these joints is rich in nerve endings and that the pain arising is often referred to the lumbar or dorsal muscles and cause much local muscle spasm. Injection of the facet joints with local anaesthetic alone or mixed with corticosteroids has had its proponents in the past. However, this is not advised as standard practice by GPs, as injection into the facet joint cavity is difficult without direct X-ray control.

Acute sciatica as a result of prolapsed intervertebral disc may be treated with epidural injection but this technique is beyond the scope of this manual.

Conditions that may be treated with local anaesthetic/steroid injections in general practice

There are often areas of localised pain in the neck, along the medial border of the scapula and in the lower lumbar spine areas that are diagnosed as 'trigger spots'. They are areas of hyperalgesia usually due to local muscle spasm and presumably arising from deeper lesions or fibromyalgia. Other more usual remedies fail to produce relief and the practitioner may often find local infiltration by injection of lidocaine 1% (1–5 ml) plain mixed with 1 ml of either triamcinolone, hydrocortisone acetate or methylprednisolone to be quite effective in providing pain relief. This treatment can be specific and only used where no other cause is demonstrable and there is no sign of nerve root irritation. Pain usually subsides after 24–48 hours and the patient frequently experiences considerable benefits.

Careful palpation of the tender area by prodding with a blunt rubber-ended probe or the finger tip will demonstrate the trigger spot, and infiltration of the whole of the lesion is necessary. The technique is similar to the injection of other soft tissue lesions such as plantar fasciitis or tennis elbow. A 10 ml syringe with a 1 inch (2.5 cm)- or a 1.5 inch (3.8 cm)-long needle is required and the injection must be given with the same careful aseptic precautions as in the other conditions described.

10 MUSCULO-SKELETAL IMAGING AND THERAPEUTIC OPTIONS IN SOFT TISSUE DISORDERS

10 MUSCULOSKELETAL IMAGING AND THERAPEUTIC OPTIONS IN SOFT TISSUE DISORDERS

David Silver

Introduction

The content of this manual has so far concentrated on the clinical diagnosis and management of soft tissue and joint disorders. Soft tissue complaints are extremely common in general practice consultations, and shoulder pain alone is a common complaint, with a reported prevalence of 6.9–34% in the general population and 21% in those over 70 years of age. It accounts for 1.2% of all general practice encounters. Uncertainty remains regarding the relative merits and efficacy for all available therapies, with little in the way of evidence-based practice available.

Training has traditionally focused on history taking, examination and clinical diagnosis, and this remains the mainstay of patient management in soft tissue disorders. Over the past decade the imaging of soft tissue and joint disorders has progressed dramatically with the advent of magnetic resonance imaging (MRI) and, more latterly, ultrasound. This has led to a significant change in the understanding of musculoskeletal disorders and the underlying biomechanical derangement. This added information can therefore be translated into clinically oriented problem solving, allowing confident diagnosis and effective management strategies, which will benefit patients in terms of treatment, prevention and effective management beyond the primary care setting. Imaging allows thinking to progress and exploration of the 'cause of the cause', i.e. the underlying biomechanical disorder. Given that soft tissue and joint disorders account for a significant proportion of consultations in general practice and hospital outpatient clinics, this part of training is sadly neglected at undergraduate and postgraduate levels.

Pathophysiology

An understanding of the pathophysiology and biomechanics of tendon disorders is fundamental to diagnosis and treatment. Imaging has led to greater knowledge and understanding of these disorders, allowing a more critical approach to their diagnosis and treatment. It should be stressed, however, that despite the power of complex imaging to demonstrate subtle tendon abnormalities, the appropriate imaging strategy and the significance of findings may not always be clear.

The terminology for tendon disorders has been confused in the past.

- *Tendinitis* is a misnomer, as inflammatory cells are rarely seen histologically.
- *Tendinopathy* is a clinical description referring to both acute and chronic conditions.
- *Tendinosis* refers to a non-inflammatory state with histological evidence of collagen disorganisation and necrosis.

Tendons without a synovial sheath, i.e. Achilles and plantar fascia, are surrounded by loose areolar tissue lined with synovial cells. This covering is called the paratenon; hence when inflamed it is called *paratenonitis*. Where a double synovial sheath is present, i.e. the tendons of the hands and feet, inflammation is referred to as *synovitis* (*see* Figure 10.1).

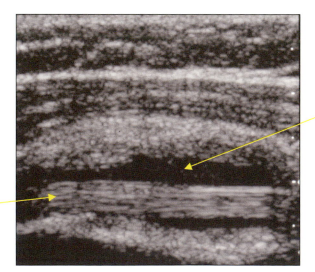

Synovial fluid

Tendon

Figure 10.1 Tenosynovitis.

The aetiology of tendinosis is multifactorial and commonly related to repeated episodes of microtrauma, with breakdown of collagen cross-linking. If repair is incomplete, it may progress to further injury and tendon failure. This theory is supported by imaging the Achilles tendon of asymptomatic athletes, where before rupture there was a history of contralateral rupture. Features in keeping with tendinosis were found in 90–95% of asymptomatic contralateral tendons. This suggests that tendon abnormalities exist that predispose to failure, thereby influencing the clinical management required to prevent further damage.

Steroid injections have been implicated as a risk factor in tendon rupture but it is not possible to distinguish between tendons that have been injected and those that have not, either radiologically or pathologically. Therefore, while cortisone in itself may not pose a risk, its anti-inflammatory effect and role as a pain reliever may lead to the overloading of degenerate tendons. It is, however, considered unwise to inject directly into a tendon as the pressure effect may lead to hypoxia and degeneration.

The underlying biomechanical disorder can be deduced from the imaging findings in abnormal tendons – the Achilles tendon is a good example where the distribution of abnormality within the tendon depends on the underlying problem, i.e. deep and medial with hyperpronation (*see* Figure 10.2), and superficial with high heel tabs. This information can be useful when prescribing corrective and preventative measures, i.e. treating the cause of the cause.

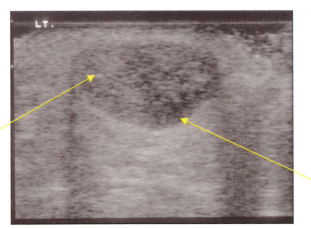

Normal tendon with echogenic appearance

Echo-poor tendinosis in deep and medial aspect

Figure 10.2 Transverse view of the Achilles tendon.

When to image

Injection techniques have been described in the previous chapters and the aim of this section is to add a further dimension to clinical practice. Not all practitioners will have confidence in making a precise diagnosis, addressing the underlying biomechanical disorder and treating it by way of advice or injection. In many instances, presentation may be 'atypical' and patients often request confirmation and traditional radiographic evidence. The use of plain film radiography in soft tissue diagnosis is limited because of the levels of radiation (levels that current European guidelines are trying to reduce). The imaging method of choice for soft tissue diagnosis is therefore either MRI or ultrasound, the latter of which carries no radiation burden. Advances in diagnostic ultrasound and its role in the resolution of soft tissue disorders means that it is now considered at least equal to or superior to MRI. It is also quicker to perform and less expensive.

As the popularity of sport and increased patient awareness of diagnostic and treatment options has led to increased demands on clinical practitioners, the option to image, with the added benefit of image-guided therapy, is now widely available to practitioners. While the majority of soft tissue disorders are either self-limiting or respond to conservative measures, including steroid injection, there are many instances where the diagnosis is unclear or the resolution of symptoms incomplete. Imaging strategies therefore offer an option for guidance without the need for traditional referral to orthopaedic clinics, whose main role is to identify surgical options.

Imaging modalities

X-rays

Plain film radiographs have an important role in demonstrating bone disorders of the shoulder, i.e. end-stage cuff arthropathy (*see* Figure 10.3), or showing erosive arthropathy (*see* Figure 10.4), but have only a minor role in imaging soft tissue and tendon abnormalities. A good example is the 'heel spur' (*see* Figure 10.5). X-ray request is no longer considered justifiable in this case, as the presence or absence of a spur bears little relationship to associated plantar fasciitis, which is directly responsible for the pain. The spur is probably secondary to the underlying biomechanical disorder.

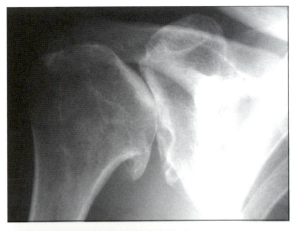

Figure 10.3 Degenerative change secondary to rotator cuff failure: 'cuff arthropathy'.

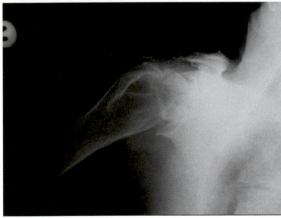

Figure 10.4 Rheumatoid arthritis of the shoulder showing erosions and destruction of the joint.

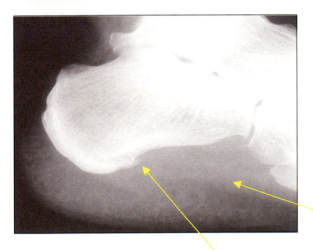

Figure 10.5 Calcaneal 'heel spur': often incidental but associated with seronegative arthropathy and Reiter's syndrome.

Plantar fascia

Inferior spur

Magnetic resonance imaging

MRI is widely used to image tendon and soft tissue pathology because the procedure avoids ionising radiation, and while there is little doubt that MRI is a powerful tool, it is expensive, time consuming and not readily available. Requests for MRI are often best discussed with a musculoskeletal radiologist prior to referral, so that the appropriateness of the study and the best way of imaging the clinical problem can be achieved. Although well established for procedures such as rotator cuff imaging (*see* Figure 10.6), MRI has been superceded to a degree by modern ultrasound techniques.

Ultrasound

Advances in probe technology over the past 15 years have revolutionised the applications of ultrasound to the imaging of smaller structures in the near field, with spatial and contrast resolution now both at least as good as, or even better than, MRI. While most radiology departments are well equipped with ultrasound equipment, the equipment for musculoskeletal imaging has to be of the highest available standard with suitable high-frequency linear array probes. The equipment is also highly dependent on operator skill.

Advantages include the ability to image in real time, hence visualising abnormalities during painful movements. A good example is shoulder impingement, which has traditionally been a clinical diagnosis but can now be confirmed with dynamic scanning.

Ultrasound offers the opportunity for image-guided intervention (*see* Figure 10.7) and is used for biopsy, aspiration of fluid from synovial swellings or joints and direct placement of steroid and local anaesthetic into tendon sheaths and bursae where there is imaging evidence of abnormality.

Relative merits for different imaging modalities

Table 10.1 summarises the relative merits of the different imaging modalities.

Imaging of joints

General principles

Having decided to refer for imaging, it is helpful to provide the radiologist with a full clinical history and examination – he can then advise on the appropriate imaging modality and provide a report, which has maximum benefit to the general practitioner (GP) or clinician in assessing further management. It is often helpful for the practitioner to see an ultrasound scan performed so that he/she can understand the technique and appreciate its strengths and weaknesses.

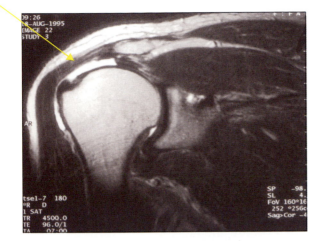

Figure 10.6 MRI: full-thickness tear of the supraspinatus.

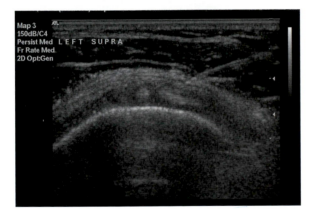

Figure 10.7 Ultrasound-guided injection of the subdeltoid bursa: note how thin the bursa is.

Table 10.1 Relative merits of different imaging modalities			
	MRI	Ultrasound	X-ray
Bone	++	+	+++
Soft tissues	+++	++++	+
Guided injection	+	+++	+
Dynamic examination	+	++++	+
Cost	++++	+	+
Length of examination	++++	+	+

It also provides an opportunity for revision of applied anatomy and pathophysiology of soft tissue disorders.

Before describing some practical examples it should be stressed that all tendons have similar appearances on ultrasound examination, and general principles relating to abnormal appearances are similar at many sites. Ultrasound images presented in this chapter represent a 'snapshot' in time and are merely a record of a dynamic and interactive procedure.

The shoulder

The aetiology of rotator cuff tears is still debated but it is primarily linked to advancing age. Other factors include impingement, deficiencies in collagen, relative avascularity and previous trauma. Shoulder pain is very common in clinical practice and patients present with a painful arc, radiation and, classically, night pain. There may be a history of trauma which is often trivial in the elderly, and typically there is little response to physiotherapy, rest or injection if there is a rotator cuff tear.

The underlying disorder may be impingement associated with micro-instability in the younger age group or more likely a rotator cuff tear with increasing age, which almost always affects the supraspinatus. Subacromial bursitis is relatively rare unless there is an underlying seropositive arthropathy with synovial proliferation, and the presence of fluid on aspiration of the bursa should point to the presence of an underlying cuff tear. The intact cuff acts as a seal between the glenohumeral joint and the subdeltoid bursa, and will therefore only distend in the presence of underlying cuff failure.

Time, rest and anti-inflammatories are the first-line treatments; only then should injections of local anaesthetic and steroid be considered.

The use of ultrasound in diagnosing impingement and rotator cuff tears is well established and is probably superior to MRI as it has the added advantage of dynamic testing and facilitates guided injections.

Lack of response to a single injection may signify an underlying tear, an incorrectly placed injection or a diagnosis that will not respond to subacromial injection. Ultrasound can be very useful in establishing the diagnosis in these cases and allows appropriate further management to be considered. With regard to rotator cuff tears, ultrasound will confirm impingement, distinguish partial from full-thickness tears and measure the size of full-thickness tears – this will have a direct impact on surgical planning. The term 'frozen shoulder' has been loosely applied in the past and this disorder is quite unusual in clinical practice. The history of pain is important, as it tends to limit all movement but pain typically presents on initiation of external rotation. Imaging is usually normal and the underlying problem relates to adhesive capsulitis, particularly involving the rotator interval between the biceps and the leading edge of the supraspinatus. Treatment options include distension arthrography to break down capsular adhesions, or manipulation under anaesthesia. Interestingly, the abnormal tissue within the rotator interval is very similar histologically to Dupytren's contracture (*see* Figures 10.8–10.15).

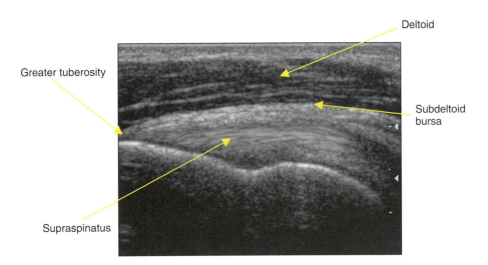

Figure 10.8 Ultrasound: normal supraspinatus (longitudinal).

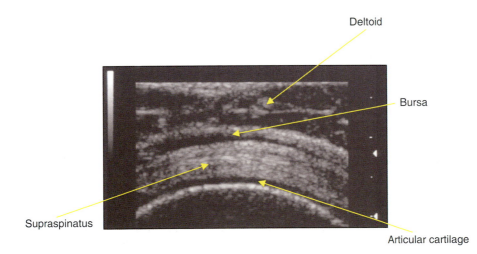

Figure 10.9 Ultrasound: normal supraspinatus (transverse).

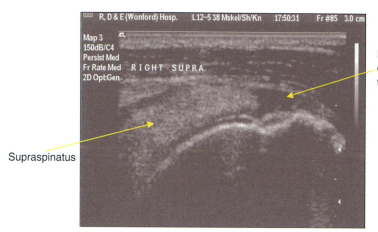

Supraspinatus

Fluid filled
defect in
tendon

Figure 10.10 Ultrasound: full-thickness tear.

'Concavity' with bursa in defect

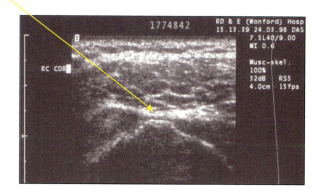

Figure 10.11 Full-thickness tear of the supraspinatus.

As the shoulder is clinically challenging, imaging has the following benefits:

- it excludes osteoarthritis
- it excludes inflammatory arthritis
- it allows diagnosis of rotator cuff tears
- it can measure the size of the tear
- it excludes biceps dislocation
- it excludes calcific tendinitis
- it allows the diagnosis of occult fractures.

Deltoid sitting on humeral head: absent supraspinatus

Bursa apposed to humeral head

Articular cartilage

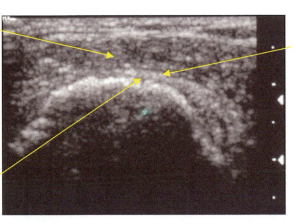

Figure 10.12 Massive rotator cuff tear.

Free margin of torn supraspinatus

Fluid filled subacromial bursa

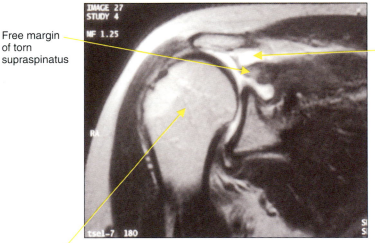

Upward subluxation of humeral head

Figure 10.13 MRI: complete tear of the supraspinatus.

Achilles tendon

The Achilles tendon is the most frequently injured ankle tendon, with injuries commonly occurring in a zone of relative avascularity 2–6 cm from the calcaneal insertion. Clinical diagnosis of complete rupture is usually straightforward.

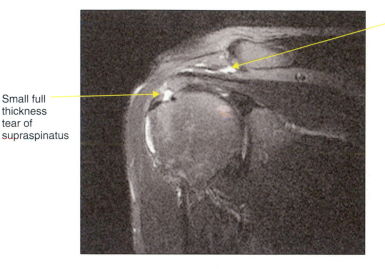

Fluid in subacromial bursa confirming full thickness tear

Small full thickness tear of supraspinatus

Figure 10.14 MRI arthrogram.

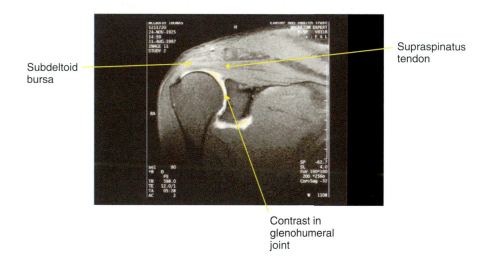

Supraspinatus tendon

Subdeltoid bursa

Contrast in glenohumeral joint

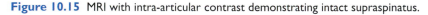

Figure 10.15 MRI with intra-articular contrast demonstrating intact supraspinatus.

Histologically, degenerative changes are present in a high percentage of spontaneous ruptures.

Ultrasound is a reliable method for imaging the abnormal Achilles tendon and with complete rupture the diagnosis can be confirmed and the distraction gap measured, which is useful in the operative assessment (*see* Figure 10.16). Plantaris tendon can be identified, which, if present, can lead to false-negative clinical tests for complete rupture. Following conservative or surgical management, ultrasound is useful for following the healing process and detecting complications.

Chronic Achilles pathology is more of a clinical challenge and ultrasound will distinguish tendinosis, partial tear and chronic rupture (*see* Figure 10.17). Metabolic disease is quite common and intratendinous gouty tophi may be identified as a cause of pain, therefore allowing appropriate management.

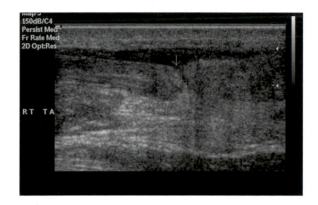

Figure 10.16 Complete tear of the Achilles tendon with fluid in the paratenon.

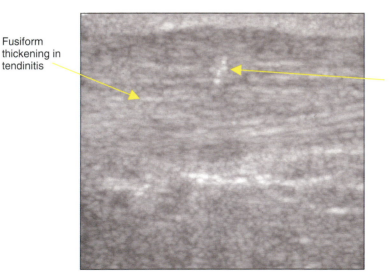

Fusiform thickening in tendinitis

Calcification seen following partial intrasubstance tearing

Figure 10.17 Longitudinal view of the Achilles tendon.

The distribution of abnormality within the tendon allows a biomechanical understanding. Superficial changes associated with a pre-Achilles bursa 'pump–bump' suggest friction between the calcaneus and high heel tabs – Haglund's disease.

Deep and medial tendinosis suggests hyperpronation, and deep and superficial tendinosis suggests muscle imbalance with abnormal loading.

The ankle

The static stabilisers, i.e. medial and lateral ligaments, are poorly visible on ultrasound and injuries are usually managed without the need to image, unless symptoms persist. The dynamic stabilisers (peroneal and medial complex) are more clearly visible. The tibialis posterior is prone to significant degeneration, and complete ruptures are frequently overlooked.

The sequel of untreated rupture includes pes planus, hindfoot valgus, forefoot abduction and midtarsal degeneration. Tears usually occur around the medial malleolus or at the navicular insertion and cause medial ankle pain, pes planus and an inability to perform a single heel raise. Diagnosis is clearly important in order to prevent long-term disability (*see* Figures 10.18 and 10.19).

Partial tears may be traumatic or secondary to tibial osteophyte formation. Not uncommonly there is a contralateral pes planus deformity, leading to overload on the affected side. Both ultrasound and MRI are useful tools in depicting tibialis tendinopathy and tears, thereby allowing early referral before rupture occurs.

Ultrasound-guided injection can be effective in treating symptoms of tibialis posterior tendinitis, allowing accurate steroid placement into the tendon sheath and avoiding tendon injection where early tenosynovitis is clinically undetectable.

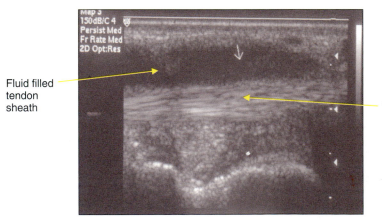

Fluid filled tendon sheath

Tendon

Figure 10.18 Tibialis posterior: tenosynovitis.

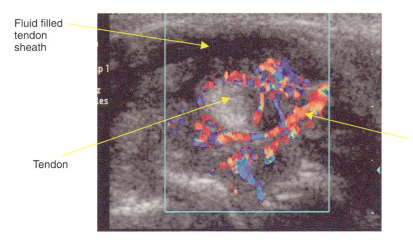

Fluid filled
tendon
sheath

Tendon

Hyperaemia
demonstrated
with colour flow
doppler

Figure 10.19 Tibialis posterior: tenosynovitis.

Plantar fascia

Inferior heel pain is a common clinical presentation and is usually due to plantar fasciitis. Inferior calcaneal bone spurs are common but are not a cause of plantar fasciitis. Ultrasound is an objective method for confirming the diagnosis. The plantar fascia will become thickened, measuring more than 0.4 cm, with decreased reflectivity from oedema and thickening of the paratenon (*see* Figure 10.20). The paratenonitis is probably responsible for the pain, so it is logical to inject this area rather than the tendon itself, which would run the risk of rupture. Ultrasound is an effective method for injecting the paratenon with steroid (which is difficult without image guidance as it is a very thin structure lying just

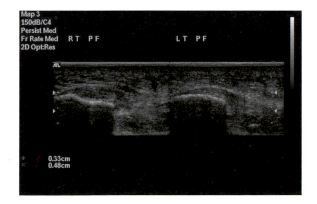

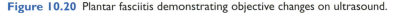

Figure 10.20 Plantar fasciitis demonstrating objective changes on ultrasound.

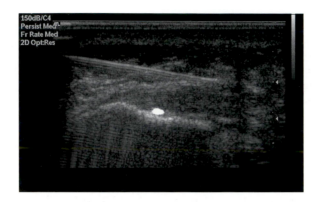

Figure 10.21 Ultrasound-guided injection of the paratenon around the plantar fascia.

superficial to the tendon), and is an effective treatment for recalcitrant fasciitis (*see* Figure 10.21).

The knee

MRI has an established role in, and is highly sensitive to detecting meniscal and cruciate injury. Ultrasound is more limited, mainly because of the depth of structures – however, it is useful in diagnosing meniscal and parameniscal abnormality and is an effective tool in examining the patellar tendon. In some cases of patellar tendinitis, there is cystic change which is unlikely to settle with conservative management; therefore, appropriate orthopaedic referral should be considered.

Ultrasound in inflammatory disease

Ultrasound has been described as 'the rheumatologist's extended finger', emphasising its extended role in the clinical examination of musculoskeletal injury or disease. As there is no associated radiation, there is no limit to the number of examinations that can be performed. It has also been demonstrated to detect erosive changes earlier than conventional radiographs. Although proven to be as effective in this regard and capable of imaging areas that are inaccessible to ultrasound (e.g. the spine and sacroiliac joints), MRI is limited in terms of availability and cost.

The potential applications of ultrasound include:

- the examination of deep joints, i.e. the hip and shoulder
- the detection of mild synovitis where clinical signs are absent

- distinction from synovitis and other causes of swelling, including tenosynovitis and subcutaneous oedema
- quantative assessment of synovitis
- differentiation between synovial hypertrophy and effusion, allowing decisions regarding aspiration to be made
- needle placement for therapeutic injection, aspiration and biopsy.

Ultrasound-guided injection

Ultrasound-guided injection allows accurate injection into proven areas of abnormality. The needle tip is visible throughout the course of the examination, which allows a single and accurate passage into a bursa, small joint or paratenon. As the undistended subacromial space measures less than 2 mm in width, accurate injection without guidance is difficult. Scanning during blind injections often shows the needle located within muscle or a tendon, with little resistance to injection.

The advantages of ultrasound-guided injection include quick and easy injection, the avoidance of multiple injections where there is lack of response, and the certainty of accurate placement. There is little evidence to suggest that either a blind or guided injection confers any advantage, but this is the subject of current research.

Calcific tendinitis

Calcific tendinitis is a painful condition that can affect any tendon, although the supraspinatus tendon of the rotator cuff is the most commonly involved. The aetiology is unclear, although repetitive trauma, a genetic predisposition or biochemical disorder, have all been implicated. Calcific deposits are common incidental findings and are thought to be painful during periods of formation and resorption. Patients often present with severe pain affecting all movements, which does not respond to local injection or anti-inflammatory drugs. While the diagnosis is commonly overlooked, once suspected it can be confirmed with radiography or ultrasound. Ultrasound is useful in confirming that the pain is attributable to the deposit and not impingement or a cuff tear. While the condition is often self-limiting, a significant number of patients will have a protracted course and further therapy should be considered.

Arthroscopic excision is a proven treatment but it does carry all the attendant risks of surgery and anaesthesia, together with a long recovery period.

A percutaneous treatment is available, which involves puncturing the deposit with two 20G needles inserted under ultrasound or fluoroscopic guidance. The procedure is performed under local anaesthesia and is well tolerated. Following multiple punctures, saline is washed through the deposit to remove some of the broken particles. Following the procedure, both steroid and Marcain® are instilled before needle removal. The procedure takes about 15 minutes to perform and is sometimes followed by a 24-hour period of exacerbation of symptoms, with a marked improvement over the next few days. The procedure is thought to produce local hyperaemia, which aids resorption of the calcific deposits. Success has been reported in up to 90% of patients who have been recalcitrant to other methods of treatment, and where symptoms have lasted for many months (*see* Figure 10.22).

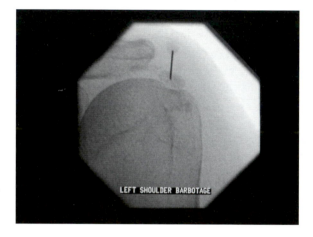

Figure 10.22 Calcific tendinitis: barbotage.

Shockwave therapy

Extracorporeal shockwave therapy (ESWL), more commonly known as lithotripsy, has been available for some time and is a well-established and effective method for treating renal calculi. It also has an established role in treating bony and soft tissue disorders, with clinical improvement of symptoms in the following areas:

- bony non-union
- calcific tendinitis
- tennis and golfer's elbow
- trochanteric bursitis
- patella tendinitis
- Achilles tendinitis
- plantar fasciitis
- Peyronie's disease of the penis.

ESWL directs shockwaves directly on to the affected tendon through ultrasound or X-ray guidance, and uses high-energy, accurately focused beams of ultrasound waves. The mechanism of action is not entirely clear but it can induce a local hyperaemic response, have an effect on cell membranes, alter the threshold of pain receptors or release negative ions, all of which are claimed to be responsible for its therapeutic response. ESWL is not widely available in the UK, and there is greater experience of its use in the USA and mainland Europe. It has clear advantages in that it has no significant side-effects, is non-invasive, and does not involve the use of steroids. Results from those centres with wide experience of its use are encouraging and are the subject of ongoing research. Current European guidelines suggest its use in refractory tendinopathy, where there has been ineffective first-line therapy, including anti-inflammatory drugs, local steroid injection and physiotherapy.

Educational aspects of reporting

It will be difficult for practising clinicians to familiarise themselves with all the complex imaging and interventional techniques now available, but as requests are made and feedback is obtained, individual referrers will begin to develop a deeper understanding of the pathology and biomechanics of common soft tissue disorders. Through this process, clinicians will become more confident in their clinical management and recognise that there may be a reason why a problem has not improved with conservative management or injection. Imaging is also a useful tool for the practitioner, allowing prompt diagnosis and effective management, leading to patient and doctor satisfaction.

Resource implications

The availability of imaging modalities and therapeutic options varies geographically, so it is up to the clinical practitioner to make the most of what is available locally. Clinicians should develop a good relationship with the providers in secondary care, who can then adapt their facilities to provide the best possible service to both patients and their doctors.

Summary

Ultrasound and MRI can be used effectively to diagnose and treat a wide range of musculoskeletal conditions. The examples in this chapter are not exhaustive but have been chosen to illustrate the role of imaging and guided therapy in some of the more common soft tissue disorders. Imaging can be used to complement clinical diagnosis and injection techniques, allowing the practitioner to become more confident in his/her diagnosis and management of soft tissue disorders.

Further reading

Blei CL *et al* (1986) Achilles tendon: ultrasound diagnosis of pathological conditions. *Radiology*. **159**: 765–7.

Bunker TD and Schranz PJ (1988) *Clinical Challenges in Orthopaedics: the shoulder*. Oxford University Press, Oxford.

Cunnane G, Brophy DP and Gibney RG (1996) Diagnosis and treatment of heel pain in chronic inflammatory arthritis using ultrasound. *Semin Arthritis Rheum*. **25**: 383–9.

Da Cruz DJ *et al* (1988) Achilles paratenonitis: an evaluation of steroid injection. *Br J Sports Med*. **22**(2): 64–5.

Farin PU and Jaroma H (1995) Acute traumatic tears of the rotator cuff: value of sonography. *Radiology*. **197**(1): 269–73.

Farin PU, Jaroma H and Soimakallio S (1995) Rotator cuff calcifications: treatment with US-guided technique. *Radiology*. **195**: 841–3.

Farin PU, Rasanen H, Jaroma H and Harju A (1996) Rotator cuff calcifications: treatment with ultrasound-guided percutaneous needle aspiration and lavage. *Skeletal Radiol*. **25**: 551–4.

Gibbon WW *et al* (1999) Sonographic incidence of tendon microtears in athletes with chronic Achilles tendinosis. *Br J Sports Med*. **33**(2): 129–30.

Green S *et al* (2001) Interventions for shoulder pain. *Cochrane Database Syst Rev* (**2**): CD001156.

Hollister MS, Mack LA and Patten RM (1995) Association of sonographically detected subacromial/subdeltoid bursal effusion and intra-articular fluid with rotator cuff tear. *Am J Roentgenol*. **165**: 605–8.

Kane D, Greaney T, Bresnihan B *et al* (1998) Ultrasound guided injection of recalcitrant plantar fasciitis. *Ann Rheum Dis*. **57**(12): 749–50.

Loew M, Daecke W, Kusnierczak D *et al* (1999) Shock-wave therapy is effective for chronic tendinitis of the shoulder. *J Bone Joint Surg Br*. **81**(5): 863–7.

Manger B and Kalden J (1995) Joint and connective tissue ultrasonography: a rheumatological bedside procedure? *Arthritis Rheum*. **38**: 736–42.

Rompe JD, Burger R, Hopf C and Eysel P (1998) Shoulder function after extracorporal shock wave therapy for calcific tendinitis. *J Shoulder Elbow Surg*. **7**: 505–9.

Rompe JD, Rumler F, Hopf C *et al* (1995) Extracorporal shock wave therapy for calcifying tendinitis of the shoulder. *Clin Orthop*. **321**: 196–201.

11 OUR PHILOSOPHY: THE BODY IS A MIRROR OF THE MIND

11 OUR PHILOSOPHY: THE BODY IS A MIRROR OF THE MIND

David MacLellan

The aim of musculoskeletal chartered physiotherapists is to return normal motor control movement, and so return the patient to normal function, whether it is sit–stand movements, or throwing the javelin at the Olympics.

This chapter aims to define sports physiotherapy and repetitive strain injuries; this is a large area to cover but the basic principles will be presented.

Physiotherapy: the history

Many physiotherapists started training as remedial gymnasts and subsequently qualified as chartered physiotherapists, as a result of amalgamation of the two professions in 1987.

Physiotherapy comes from a nursing/medical model, and remedial gymnastics came from a physical training instructor, movement/exercise background. The two disciplines' societies merged in 1987 and the professional status became 'chartered physiotherapists'.

It has been suggested within the profession that the movement aspect and rehabilitation base was not being taught and that instead we concentrated on electrotherapy and focused on micromanagement of conditions.

Physiotherapists have a broader or holistic view of movement and how maladaptive it can be. It is now considered that physiotherapists as a profession are beginning to regain some of those lost ideas, and are again beginning to lead the way; the term 'functional rehab' has become one of the professions' 'buzz' phrases.

There is a greater evidence base now available as a result of significant research in the field of physiotherapy, which has dramatically raised the profile of this important aspect of management of musculoskeletal disorders.

What do physiotherapists do?

Musculoskeletal physiotherapists are closely involved with patient's experiences and colleagues' continuous professional development, whether in the private or public healthcare setting or in sports teams, which shapes and hones the treatment ethos for our patients.

Physiotherapists are experts in their field – we assess, diagnose, treat and work within a dynamic multidisciplinary team.

It is key to listen to what the patient/athlete is saying; they may not verbalise exactly what we expect to hear, but they will generally lead the physiotherapist to a primary impression of what is wrong, whatever it may be – traumatic/subacute/repetitive or pathology based.

- Watch how they move, as this will generally give you very valuable non-verbal clues.
- Be precise with your testing; try to ensure that your tests are sensitive and specific.
- Make your diagnosis, and keep the message/information simple for your patient/athlete to understand.

The major difference between you and I and the elite athlete is talent. Please remember that you are in a similar position – you just won't win a medal if you make the correct diagnosis and your patients get better.

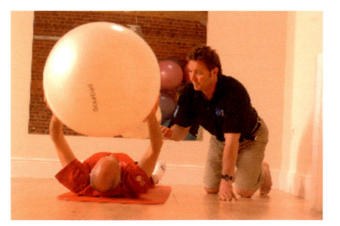

Figure 11.1 Shoulder rehab with increased sensory input. Gravity assisted.

WHY? I have a feeling that this is something to do with the fact that physio-therapy has been a guru-led profession. This may sound somewhat degrading to these 'gurus' – not in the least. They are in fact clinicians who have made us think and have given us direction over these last 10–15 years. The profession is growing up quite quickly at present and I feel that this leads us to ensuring that most of our work is based on evidence from clinical researchers.

This has put a biopsychosocial perspective on some of our more chronic patients, and often these people are maladapters. This may be due to pain, which can be a severe and negative experience, leading to pain avoidance and fear, and possibly ultimately resulting in disability and depression. Motor control is regained and normal function returned by ensuring that any adaptations to pain are assessed and corrected. Of course, other methods are also used, such as ice, electrother-apy, soft tissue massage, joint manipulation and exercise, to name a few. They are all utilised at the optimal time for that pathology or condition.

I feel that, as a profession, we had become too focused on the micromanagement, without looking at the whole picture. This is not to say that the microstructures are not important, there is no point in having a well-healed ankle ligament if the patient has now got non-specific back pain, due to their maladaption – which is where the author's and co-authors' experience comes in.

Sports injuries

A significant factor in sports injuries is that other people witness the incident. This is where immediate care of an acute sports injury, whether it be a sprain, tear, rupture or worse, can be managed early and well. Immediate care can def-initely minimise the damage to soft tissue and can save days and sometimes weeks of an athlete's treatment and rehabilitation phase. This is not something that most patients have access to.

Example: anterior talofibular ligament sprain grade 1

You or I may decide we can walk on that grade 1 ankle sprain; are we making it worse? We are certainly not helping the natural response, which is pain and inflammation – Mother Nature's first aid.

This leads us to ongoing adaptive movement patterns; do we adapt to the pain? Most of us will limp for a few days depending on our perception of pain; however, this could go on longer and we start to maladapt in terms of our movement patterns, i.e. start to load other structures such as the hip and back. It is not uncommon to see patients three weeks or so down the line who are experiencing back pain.

In sport-specific injuries, the physiotherapist works very hard to prevent maladaptive movement, so those first few hours are very important.

In our practice we see a lot of patients with maladaptive patterns of movement throughout the body, whether through initial trauma or as a result of repetitive injuries.

To prevent these maladaptive patterns and gain the correct motor control, it is important to understand and interpret movement behaviours, in order to reduce or eliminate the pain, effusion, swelling or spasm that is over-protecting and creating this maladaptive pattern.

- Motor control describes the way a task is performed – it is not a muscle contraction.
- If a movement or posture has changed this is altered motor control.
- No muscles work in isolation.
- The brain works at performing the task – not contracting a muscle.
- The brain learns movement by task orientation and practice.

LISTEN . . . . WATCH . . . . KEEP IT PRECISE AND SIMPLE.

Adapters and maladapters

Motor control responses may be adaptive or maladaptive. To perform a task, a balance should be maintained between maximal efficiency and protecting the musculoskeletal system and the body's physiological process.

- *Adaptive motor control*: movement behaviour is pain protective.
- *Maladaptive motor control*: a task is performed in a manner that results in compromising of the musculoskeletal system and/or the body's physiological processes. Maladaptive motor control/movement/ cognitive behaviours are provocative of the pain disorder.

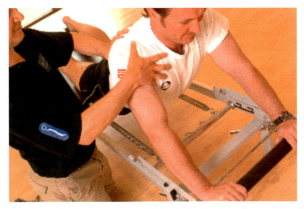

Figure 11.2 Specific movement patterning for a maladapter, 'spinal extension' using a pilates reformer.

Methods of treatment

Ice/cryotherapy

Some of the most recent research suggests that icing a limb or part of it should be done for 10 minutes in every half hour for 4–6 h. In our practice we use a cryotherapy and compression system called Game Ready®. It consists of a compression garment that utilises a pump to circulate cold water around the traumatised area while maintaining the pressure and temperature. We have found it to be an invaluable aid in helping to control the inflammatory stage.

Manual therapy

Every competent physiotherapist should have good handling skills, and a very precise idea of what they are feeling (palpation); this is what sets us apart from other professions. Palpation can be carried out on neural tissue or may involve using the right pressure on an effused/swollen joint that is painful.

- *Joint mobilisation*: a series of specific accessory movements created by the clinician to aid movement of a joint in a specified direction. These movements are graded 1–4, where 1 is very slight movement and 4 takes the joint structure to its end range.
- *Joint manipulation*: a final level, grade 5, requires the clinician to specifically position the patient in order to manipulate the correct level. If done well, this does not require massive force, simply good technique.
- *Soft tissue massage/mobilisation*: this involves flushing the affected soft tissue around the injured area. It can be performed very early in the care process and involves light pressure to aid venous return and reduce swelling in the early stages of tissue injury. However, there are some very powerful techniques that may be used to break down scar tissue and these can be quite painful.

Therapeutic ultrasound

This method can be used from 72 h after injury, to help the microrepair of soft tissue at cellular level.

Electrotherapy

There are many types of electrotherapy that claim to aid soft tissue repair and reduce inflammation. Most of these have their roles to play, but detailed discussion of the techniques would probably form a chapter in its own right.

Acupuncture

This ancient practice is a very useful tool in treating a wide and diverse group of patients and conditions. At times it can have quite startling results, especially for spasm and regional non-specific pain.

Movement patterning

This starts at the initial assessment, and becomes more defined as the physio-therapist spends more time with the patient. It may start with general postural advice and finish with a very specific pattern pertaining to their work or sport.

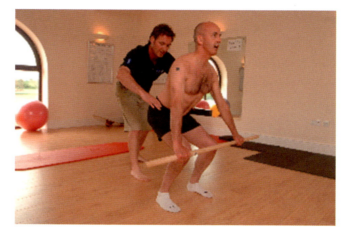

Figure 11.3 Functional movement patterning, during early stage of rehab (low loading).

Functional rehabilitation

What is the specific activity that your patient would like to return to – for example, is it tennis, gardening or work? Are you devising a programme so that your patient can go upstairs safely after having a fall, or are you ensuring that the rugby fly-half is able to kick the ball three weeks after his grade 2 anterior talo-fibular ligament (ATFL) sprain?

There are a myriad of aids for functional rehabilitation, such as wobble boards, resistance bands, etc. The challenge for the physiotherapist is to gain enough input for the patient without overloading weakened or damaged tissue structure. This takes smart clinical reasoning and assessment of the stage of repair/healing, coupled with a lot of experience and understanding of perceived normal movement. One of the best and most recognised functional tools we use within the clinical setting is pilates.

Clinical pilates

The major difference between this and the usual form of pilates is that it is clinician led, and so it is vital for the patient that the clinician understands the pathology and correct movement direction.

Its basis is well researched; it is used to unravel some long-term maladaptive movement patterns and helps restore efficiency and control to movement.

Within the profession, there is a very skilled and diligent group of practioners who are leaders in the field of clinical pilates. In many instances patients have practised pilates for a few years, occasionally in the leisure setting, but we find that the specificity of the movements has been misconstrued or that certain muscle groups have been over-recruited.

Injection therapy

There are a growing number of physiotherapists who inject clinically. However, as this book is based around the musculoskeletal injection techniques, there is no need to discuss that here.

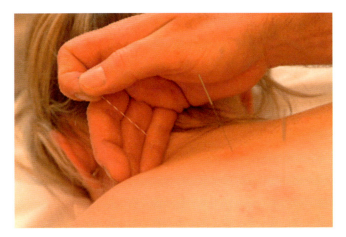

Figure 11.4 Trigger point acupuncture for over active muscle tissue. Upper trapezius and levator scapulae muscles.

How do we interact with our medical colleagues and what do we ask of them?

In our practice we work closely with primary care physicians and consultants who are forward thinking and comfortable with our ethos and practice. They are happy to work together with us for the benefit of the patient.

Physiotherapists are used primarily by two diverse groups:

- as a first port of call for soft tissue sprains and strains
- or as a specialist's ongoing referral pathway, which may be from a general practitioner (GPs) or other health care professional.

The first group generally come straight to us, without undergoing any investigations or procedures or receiving any medication, except for self-administration of first aid, and they may not need intervention. Once assessed, if further investigations are needed we send them to our local musculoskeletal radiologist for either ultrasound, magnetic resonance imaging (MRI) or X-ray, to help confirm our clinical diagnosis. This feedback from specialists is essential; it is based on many years of trust and forms part of our ongoing clinical development. As my co-author once told me, 'We treat patients not MRIs'.

Those in the second group generally arrive clutching X-rays, MRI scans or a disc that they hope will have some of the answers to their problems. It is important to have as much of their clinical information as possible in order to help the physiotherapist understand what is relevant to them and their condition, and time is often spent in the initial consultation unravelling all the perceptions or misinterpretations that the patient has gleaned on their journey.

Clinical examples

A classic example is that of a patient who comes to us with a diagnosis of tennis elbow (lateral epicondylitis).

We estimate that two out of ten patients that present or are referred do not have a true tennis elbow, i.e. they only have pain around the common extensor origin with no other symptoms. A common scenario is that the patient presents with pain around the outside of the elbow joint, that has been there for 3–4 weeks and appeared after some repetitive movements. They have not been to the GP and have taken non-steroidal anti-inflammatory drugs (NSAIDS) or some form of painkiller. They have come to see us because they are in pain and are not able to carry on with their daily activities.

These patients are assessed fully from the cervical spine down to the wrist and hand, for neural joint or myofascial related pain. If these are clear, their condition is usually a true tennis elbow.

The methods of treatment commonly used are:

- ultrasound
- soft tissue massage
- specific muscle stretching.

There is also a good case for injection therapy at this stage, to reduce the pain and allow a window to enable ongoing physiotherapy. This is when having very good and cooperative medical management is essential, to obtain a good result for the patient.

The second scenario is of a similar presentation with what appears to be an insidious onset.

This patient will start to describe varied points or areas of pain. Once these have been drawn on a body chart, it starts to become apparent that this is not a classic tennis elbow, as the patient tends to describe C5–C8 dermatomal pain, or part thereof. These pains can be vague or specific, and generally show frequent changes in severity and location. The patients will have overactive muscle around the upper fibres of the trapezius, levator scapulae and tight pectoralis minor. They will often have an elevated first rib and will be sensitive to neural testing or palpation.

They often fall into the group of work-related upper limb disorders. This type of condition can be very hard to treat and may have a significant biopsychosocial perspective. A multifaceted approach should be used, in terms of the treatment methods and clinicians involved.

The future

This chapter outlines the role of physiotherapy in soft tissue conditions; it should be stressed that this is a large area to cover, but it is hoped that the information will enlighten a few clinicians, in the not so dark arts of physiotherapy.

We are lucky in our practice that we have time and motivated patients; this is what most patients need, and has not always been their experience in the past.

Our profession needs to be constantly challenged, and so do our practices and beliefs if we are to stay at the forefront of world-class musculoskeletal research and treatment.

Further reading

Brown C (2009) Mazes, conflict, and paradox: tools for understanding chronic pain. *Pain Pract*. **9**(3): 235–43

Leeuw M *et al* (2007) The fear-avoidance model of musculoskeletal pain: current state of scientific evidence. *J Behav Med*. **30**(1): 77–94.

Moseley L (2008) Pain, brain imaging and physiotherapy – opportunity is knocking. *Man Ther*. **13**: 475–7.

O'Sullivan PB, Beales D (2007) Classification of pelvic girdle pain disorders. Part 1 with a mechanism based approach within a biopsychosocial framework. *Man Ther*. **12**(2): 86–97.

INDEX

INDEX